DATE DUE

ILL –			
SWIFT			
#36029			
San Juan			
4-24-02			

GAYLORD   PRINTED IN U.S.A

The Challenge of Fetal Alcohol Syndrome

Overcoming Secondary Disabilities

The Challenge of Fetal Alcohol Syndrome
Overcoming Secondary Disabilities

Edited by
Ann Streissguth
and
Jonathan Kanter

Foreword by
Mike Lowry

Introduction by
Michael Dorris

University of Washington Press
Seattle and London

Library of Congress Cataloging-in-Publication Data
The challenge of fetal alcohol syndrome: overcoming secondary
  disabilities / Ann P. Streissguth and Jonathan Kanter, editors; with an
  introduction by Michael Dorris.
     p. cm.
  Includes bibliographical references and index.
  ISBN 0–295–97650–0 (alk. paper)
  1. Children of prenatal alcohol abuse—Development.   2. Children of
prenatal alcohol abuse—Services for.   3. Fetal alcohol syndrome—
Complications.   I. Streissguth, Ann P.   II. Kanter, Jonathan.
RJ520.P74C46   1997   97–18618
618.3′268—dc21   CIP

The paper used in this publication meets the minimum requirements of American National Standard for Information Sciences—Permanence of Paper for Printed Library Materials, ANSI Z39.48–1984. ∞

Cover photography by George Steinmetz

Contents

Foreword

Governor Mike Lowry

I believe that research on Fetal Alcohol Syndrome (FAS) and Fetal Alcohol Effects (FAE) clearly is one of the most important issues in all the world today.

Why does a Governor care so much about FAS? First, Governors are human beings, too, and supporting this research is simply the right thing to do.

Second, every one in elected office has many good governmental reasons to care about and support efforts to find answers to this tremendous problem. For example, most of the children that become dependent on the state of Washington for support, and not on their own families, do so through Children's Protective Services or related programs. Sixty-three percent of the children who became dependent on the state of Washington in 1995 became dependent because of reasons related to substance abuse. This is not to say that 63% of children in state care were victims of FAS, but that substance abuse was the major factor in 63% of the decisions that social workers, other professionals, and judges made to have the state protect our children and remove them from their homes.

We simply have not met our very first responsibility: protection of our children. We will not meet this responsibility until we commit ourselves to finding answers to the problems of substance abuse and its effects on our children. This must be done or we must seriously question ourselves when we claim to care about our dependent children.

I am not an expert about Fetal Alcohol Syndrome. However, I have had numerous discussions with judges about some of the absolutely incomprehensible crimes that have been created and committed in this and other states, crimes committed by and against teenagers and young adults. These judges were certain that the major cause of these crimes was FAS. These judges were certain that the perpetrators of these crimes simply did not have the ability to judge what was happening around them.

The crimes perpetrated by victims of FAS are on the terrible, extreme end of a continuum of secondary effects of FAS and FAE that result in a huge cost to society. It is the job of all elected officials to respond to this problem. It is our job to identify the problems that our society faces and then work with everyone to find solutions to these problems.

A meaningful investment by the public sector in addressing these problems actually is very affordable. The Washington State budget (which I happen to know a little bit about) currently is funding a number of programs such as the Birth to 3 program, described in this volume (see chapter by Grant, Ernst, Streissguth, and Porter). This program has been shown, among other things, to be effective at preventing high-risk women from birthing fetal-alcohol affected babies. It is very well run and is very important. We could increase the funds available for this program by a factor of 25 and this would cost the average homeowner in the state of Washington 25 cents per month. Our economy currently is doing very well, and our budget is in great shape, so I am not suggesting a 25 cent per month tax increase. Rather, I am suggesting not cutting taxes by 25 cents per month. Twenty-five cents per month! Those 25 cents would go a long way.

One thing I have never understood is why the financially well-to-do are so against paying taxes. The only things their money cannot buy are the things that taxes pay for: clean air, clean water, safe streets, enlightened society. Even Bill Gates cannot buy these things. The well-to-do should be lining up in the streets demanding to pay higher taxes, so that they can achieve safety in the streets for their children and the other things that, strictly speaking, their money cannot buy. It is understandable that low and middle income people do not like taxes. But some commitments make sense. A commitment to addressing the problem of FAS makes sense.

By the year 2000 in Washington state, we will have one billion dollars more in our general fund per year than our present law allows us to spend. We will have the resources necessary to invest in human capital to support the programs and ideas, and address the problems, that are presented in this book. All we need is a political and social commitment. It is up to us as a society to come together and answer these questions.

I was delighted and proud to be a part of the conference that inspired this book. This conference, held in Seattle, Washington in 1996, drew together people from 39 states and eight countries to discuss these issues, and it demonstrated that this is a situation that we are all in together. It is a situation that forces us to ask ourselves: In what ways do we care about our society and our children?

My wife, Mary Lowry, always has been the most effective lobbyist on this particular Governor. She received information from Ann

Streissguth's Fetal Alcohol and Drug Unit and other organizations, and educated both of us about this problem. Once I learned about this problem, and realized that this is a problem that truly can be prevented, I became a strong advocate.

Now we all must become advocates. The information in this book, added to the facts already known about FAS, can make a difference. You should use this information; use it to inform legislators, governors, the news media, and all the people who are a part of our society's decision-making process. Tell them that there is only one right decision about FAS. Tell them that in order to meet the basic responsibilities of their jobs they must support the ideas and programs in this book that aim to overcome and prevent secondary disabilities in FAS and FAE. They must find answers to Fetal Alcohol Syndrome and Fetal Alcohol Effects. This is vitally important material and with it we can make a tremendous difference to many people in this world.

Preface

This book commemorates 25 years of research on Fetal Alcohol Syndrome (FAS) at the University of Washington Medical School. From the initial identification and naming of FAS in 1973, through the first international conference on FAS in 1980, the major nonhuman primate studies of FAS, and the first follow-up study of adolescents and adults with FAS, Seattle researchers have been actively involved in both research and clinical work with people with FAS and their families.

In September 1996, 653 people from 8 countries and 39 states gathered at the University of Washington Medical School to hear new research findings from the Fetal Alcohol Follow-up Study, and to hear what 62 colleagues representing many different professional backgrounds, national and community organizations, and types of families were doing to actually help people with FAS. This book contains 22 selected papers from this three-day conference, and a Rapporteur's Report summarizing the individual presentations of most of the rest of the presenters.

Fetal Alcohol Syndrome was named as a birth defect in 1973 when two University of Washington dysmorphologists (Drs. Kenneth Lyons Jones and David W. Smith) identified 11 unrelated children from three racial backgrounds with a similar pattern of craniofacial anomalies, growth deficiency, and central nervous system (CNS) dysfunction. All were born to alcoholic mothers. The news was shocking, and met at first with disbelief.

Within four years, experimental animal studies clearly established that alcohol is a teratogenic drug and a case-comparison group study was carried out showing that children of alcoholic mothers, even when compared to carefully-matched controls, have more growth deficiency, smaller head circumference, and more borderline to moderate mental retardation. By 1978, 245 patients with FAS had been reported in the medical literature, and FAS was described as the most frequent known cause of mental deficiency. Several necropsy reports on children with FAS revealed serious brain anomalies, and experimental animal studies, including a series of nonhuman primate studies carried out at the University of Washington Primate Center by Dr. Sterling Clarren and colleagues, confirmed the vulnerability of the fetal brain to prenatal alcohol exposure.

Because FAS was clearly an entirely preventable birth defect, prevention efforts were underway within a few years of the initial identification. In 1981 the Surgeon General issued a Health Warning on Alcohol and Pregnancy, recommending that women who are pregnant or considering a pregnancy refrain from alcohol use. By 1989 national legislation was passed mandating warning labels about the harmful effects of drinking during pregnancy, and many cities and states now have mandatory posting of warning signs at point of purchase of all alcohol beverages. Public awareness of the risks of drinking during pregnancy is high.

However, intervention efforts to help people with FAS and their families have not kept pace. A Dysmorphology Unit and a Craniofacial Clinic at the University of Washington Medical School and Children's Hospital and Medical Center over the years between 1973 and 1991, identified many local infants and children, either with FAS or with Fetal Alcohol Effects (FAE) or Possible Fetal Alcohol Effects (PFAE). FAE and PFAE were terms used for patients who had some but not all of the characteristics of FAS, but had a history of significant prenatal alcohol exposure. A ten-year follow-up study of the first eleven children identified with FAS revealed a surprising degree of psychosocial distress, especially in those who had the highest IQ scores. Larger studies of more adolescents and adults revealed similar findings, not only from Seattle, but from other cities and countries as well.

Further data were clearly needed to document and understand the breadth and magnitude of the problems faced by people with FAS and FAE as they grew up. In 1992, the Centers for Disease Control (CDC), through the National Center for Environmental Health, Disabilities Prevention Program, funded researchers at the University of Washington Medical School to carry out two important studies with practical significance for people with FAS/FAE and their families.

Drs. Clarren and Astley in the University of Washington Department of Pediatrics were funded to run a weekly FAS diagnostic clinic, ostensibly as a vehicle for studying birth mothers of such patients, but which actually provided the first opportunity for the systematic examination of hundreds of people of all ages born to alcohol-abusing mothers.

Our team at the Fetal Alcohol & Drug Unit in the Department of Psychiatry and Behavioral Sciences was funded to carry out a study of secondary disabilities in people with FAS/FAE. This CDC study was designed to reduce the incidence and severity of primary and secondary disabilities and to promote the independence, productivity and integration into the community of persons with disabilities. For the purpose of this current work, primary disabilities were defined as those that reflect the CNS dysfunction inherent in the FAS or FAE diagnosis. Secondary disabilities were those that a person is not born with and that could presumable be ameliorated through better understanding and appropriate interventions. The secondary disabilities under particular investigation were those that our clinical experience with hundreds of similar patients suggested were frequently a problem. They included mental health problems, disrupted school experiences, trouble with the law, inappropriate sexual behaviors, alcohol and drug abuse, difficulty with independent living, difficulty with employment, and problems with parenting. It was our hope that good descriptive data on the frequency of these secondary disabilities in people with FAS/FAE would draw attention to this problem, generate interest in understanding and responding to the needs of this population of under-served people, and stimulate further research and more effective service delivery.

In 1996 The Institute of Medicine (IOM) published a review of *Fetal Alcohol Syndrome: Diagnosis, epidemiology, prevention, and treatment* (Stratton, Howe, & Battaglia, 1996) in which a new term for FAE and PFAE was introduced: "Alcohol-Related Neurodevelopmental Disorder" (ARND). The terms FAE and PFAE as used in the papers by Clarren and colleagues and Streissguth and colleagues are interchangeable with ARND.

Because the intent of our study was to generate interest and action toward effective intervention efforts, research also was undertaken on the risk and protective factors associated with these secondary disabilities. We wanted to be able to say to communities: Here's a huge problem, but here are some things that happen to a child postnatally that are related to an increase or a decrease in this problem. Once communities have this information, they should be a giant step ahead in planning for the needs of people with FAS/FAE and their families, in ways that should specifically improve their lives.

This book, like the conference and study that inspired it, arose from the need for more information about Fetal Alcohol Syndrome (FAS) and Fetal Alcohol Effects (FAE). What do we know about the brain damage that causes FAS, what are people with FAS like, what are their predictable disabilities, and what are some promising ways of overcoming these disabilities? Thanks to substantial funding from the CDC, we are now able to move forward with information about these disabilities and the interventions that might help. This information was published in a Final Report to the CDC, but that was only our preliminary medium of dissemination. The next step was the three-day international conference "Overcoming and Preventing Secondary Disabilities in Fetal Alcohol Syndrome and Fetal Alcohol Effects" held September 4 to 6, 1996 at the University of Washington Health Sciences/Medical Center in Seattle, Washington. We thought of it not so much as a research meeting, but as a working meeting where people could learn from each other, be inspired by each other, and take ideas back to their own communities. In inviting the speakers, we sought out people from around the world who were doing something new that could have direct implications to promoting understanding and help for people with FAS/FAE in the hope of preventing and overcoming the secondary disabilities of FAS/FAE.

This book is the next step in disseminating this information. This book is for anyone who is concerned about doing something to help people with FAS/FAE and their families. There are papers describing programs and interventions from many different professionals — and from family members too — who must work together to provide the network of appropriate services for people with FAS. This book is for people in mental health, the schools, criminal and juvenile justice, politicians and government administrators and policy planners; it is also for families with the hope it will generate ideas about where to turn for help. This book is for people who want to be part of the solution, who want to be aware of the latest ideas on overcoming and preventing secondary disabilities in people with FAS/FAE. This book is for those who want to find inspiration for how to proceed in every community for the improved welfare and humane understanding of this underserved population.

The book opens, as did the conference, with a Foreword by then-Governor Mike Lowry, who truly put the weight of his office energetically behind efforts to overcome and prevent these disabilities in our state. He supported legislation about warning signs about not drinking during pregnancy and legislation to mandate an FAS coordinating committee of state executives whose activities relate to people with FAS across all branches of state government. He supported legislation to guarantee access to a network of FAS diagnostic clinics across the state, and used money from his emergency fund to set up a new program of Birth to 3, the Seattle Advocacy model for strenuous intervention with the very highest risk group of mothers. Governor Lowry set a new standard for the governors of our states. As you read his words, determine to make *your* Governor involved to the same fruitful extent.

Since 1973, FAS has been the topic of extensive research and thousands of children have been diagnosed with this birth defect.

Enormous efforts have been undertaken to get the word out about FAS. But not until 1989, with the gift of Michael Dorris's word, was that milestone finally achieved. His book, *The Broken Cord*, written with tenderness and understanding about his son with FAS, has done more than all my research to bring the reality of FAS to the public eye. In the Introduction to the present book, Michael Dorris speaks as a "parent with issues" about his son Abel, who ". . . lived for 23 years, endured daily loneliness and confusion and hardship and frustration, and in all that time never once did anything that was intentionally cruel or hurtful to another living creature." As Dorris says, "He was maddening in his inability to learn from experience, to grasp a larger picture, but he was also sweetness distilled." Dorris points out what is seldom noted, that the vast majority of people afflicted with FAS or FAE in this world are not children, but adults. And he reminds us that Fetal Alcohol Syndrome can be eliminated, "but it is a slow and painstaking process . . . one rescued human life at a time."

Drs. Sarah Mattson and Ed Riley present a scholarly review of the literature documenting the research of the past 20 years on the effects of prenatal alcohol exposure on intelligence, language, visual spatial functioning, verbal learning and memory, motor abilities, and attention. They also document research findings relating to neuro-anatomic features of FAS and FAE from the early autopsy findings to the latest imaging studies, much of the latter carried out on their patients. They conclude that prenatal alcohol exposure has pervasive and often devastating consequences to the brain, but also that there is some evidence for a specific pattern of effects in individuals with FAS and FAE.

Dr. Marita Aronson, a long-time FAS researcher, presents a summary of 25 years of research on children of alcoholic mothers in Göteborg, Sweden. She finds that although good foster homes could not fully compensate for the prenatally acquired handicap, it was her clinical impression that the fostered children were better able to cope with difficulties than were those who remained in the biologic home when the mother continued to abuse alcohol.

My colleagues and I present a summary of the CDC study, described above, primary disabilities, measured with tests of IQ, achievement and adaptive functioning, observed in the latest study of 473 people with FAS/FAE, who range in age from 3 to 51 years of age. We also present a summary of the frequency of secondary disabilities observed in a similar group of 415 patients. Specific factors associated with increased risk of secondary disabilities, as well as specific "protective" factors associated with a decreased risk of secondary disabilities that communities and families could provide are described. One of the strongest factors that protects against secondary disabilities is an early diagnosis, something still too difficult to obtain in many states and communities.

Drs. Clarren and Astley present a comprehensive report on how they developed a fetal alcohol diagnostic and prevention network in Washington State that is underway at seven sites, serving the FAS diagnostic and prevention needs of communities. This model grew out of Dr. Clarren's long experience diagnosing FAS within a medical clinic context, and his resolve to develop a new type of clinic that is responsive to the medical, psychiatric, psychologic, educational, and social needs of the patients and their parents. Developing these clinics within a community context where local professionals are involved at the outset in the diagnostic examination and recommendations means that the diagnosis leads directly to workable intervention and treatment recommendations. Experience with the first 511 patients evaluated at the UW clinic site is described as well as methods for development, funding and staffing of such statewide networks.

Chapters by Dr. Kathleen Dyer and colleagues and Jill Snyder and colleagues describe two small intervention studies with patients with FAS. The former describes a neuropsychologic and behavior modification approach, the latter a controlled medication study for patients with FAS thought to be responsive to stimulant medication.

Two chapters focus on the schools. Dr. Patricia Tanner-Halverson describes techniques developed for early intervention within the classroom setting over the past six years when she ran a demonstration classroom for young children with FAS/FAE which began with a small pilot program from the Arizona State Department of Education. Dr. Thomas Wentz presents the shocking findings from his 1995 national survey of state directors of special education in which he found, for example, that only three of the 50 states surveyed had taken any action on FAS, based on a discussion of this problem.

Two chapters discuss case management solutions for people with FAS/FAE. Claire Anita Schmucker gives specific tips on how a privately paid case manager and independent living instructor can assist patients with FAS/FAE. Therese Grant and colleagues describe how a successful model developed for the highest risk mothers in the community who are abusing alcohol and drugs during pregnancy and getting little or no prenatal care (Birth to 3: The Seattle Advocacy Model) can be adapted to meet the needs of mothers who themselves have FAS/FAE, as they face pregnancy and parenting challenges with adolescence and adulthood.

Three chapters are by two lawyers and a judge who have success-fully advocated for young adults with FAS. Peter McKee, in plain language, describes the ins and outs of the social security system from the standpoint of an FAS client. Jeanice Dagher-Margosian describes her defense of a client with FAS in a criminal case and the relevance of the FAS diagnosis to each phase of the criminal investi-gation. The Honorable C. C. Barnett, whose powerful utilization of FAS as a sentencing factor in *Regina vs. Rose Abou* inspired the work of Dagher-Margosian in her sentencing appeal, describes how he reached his decision that it is "simply obscene to suggest that a court can properly warn other potential offenders by inflicting a form of punishment upon a handicapped person who has, indeed, commit-ted an offense for which some sanction must follow." He describes how he used sentencing to focus on some measure of protection for others and to provide a realistic framework for rehabilitation for the offender herself.

Two chapters are written by psychologists involved in various ways with adolescents and adults with FAS and FAE. Dr. Robin LaDue and Tom Dunne, M.S.W. review FAS evaluations for legal determina-tion of competency, capacity, diminished capacity, decline/remand, and highlight problems in making each determination. Dr. Natalie Novick describes treatment issues with sexual offenders diagnosed with FAS, and offers advice to parents on coping strategies at home to prevent inappropriate sexual behaviors from reaching the level of a criminal offense.

In two chapters, parents describe their special contributions to preventing and overcoming secondary disabilities in FAS/FAE. Jocie DeVries and Ann Waller describe their effective efforts for public policy change for increased services for people with FAS/FAE in Washington state, and their successful mobilization of a parent support network for political action. Jan Lutke, with 20 years' experi-ence raising children with FAS/FAE, describes how she has learned from her children the practical meaning of problems with memory, motivation, and time — "spider web walking" as her daughter describes it.

Finally, three administrators approach FAS from a more global perspective. Joseph Hess M.S.W., M.B.A., and Dr. George Nieman describe residential programs needed in the community to meet the continuum of care and comprehensive service needs of people with FAS/FAE. Richard Jackson, M.D., Director of CDC's National Center for Environmental Health, approaches FAS from a public health standpoint. He reviews other toxicants, such as lead, that damage developing brains, which have seen a dramatic decline over the past two decades as a result of changes in general knowledge and public policy, and compares these problems to FAS. From a public health standpoint, the best intervention is prevention.

In the final chapter, Fred Bookstein, who took copious notes throughout the three days of the conference, presents in his "Rapporteur's Report" pithy summaries of the presentations of thirty additional speakers.

As it goes to press, this book is dedicated with great admiration and sorrow to Michael Dorris, whose untimely death on 11 April 1997 stilled our most passionate voice for FAS.

Ann Streissguth
April 1997
Seattle, Washington

Acknowledgments

This book began with a conference, which began with a research grant, which was made possible by four years of funding from the Centers for Disease Control (CDC; Grant Number R04/CCR008515). The special support of four people at CDC is gratefully acknowledged Richard Jackson, M.D., Director of the National Center for Environmental Health (NCEH), the funding source for the research; Godfrey P. Oakley, Jr., M.D., Director, Division of Birth Defects and Developmental Disabilities, always a strong voice for the importance of applied research on this very prevalent birth defect; Karen Hymbaugh, M.P.A., M.P.H., NCEH Developmental Disabilities Branch, technical consultant on this research, always a dependable source of good judgment and advice; and Joe Smith, our Project Officer at NCEH whose unfailing enthusiasm and personal commitment to this work is greatly appreciated.

Thanks are due to many who made the conference on "Overcoming and Preventing Secondary Disabilities in Fetal Alcohol Syndrome and Fetal Alcohol Effects" such a success Pam Phipps, Research Manager of our Fetal Alcohol & Drug Unit (FADU) was the mainstay of organization and innovation; Jonathan Kanter, M.A., with exquisite attention to detail, was the Conference Coordinator. A Community Steering Committee, made up of local colleagues passionate about FAS education (Jocie DeVries, Co-Director of the FAS Family Resource Institute; Therese Grant, Ph.C., FADU; Louise Harper, M.A., Bellevue; Robin LaDue, Ph.D., FADU and Private Practice, Seattle; Sandra Randels, M.S.N., past Washington State FAS Coordinator; and Marceil TenEyck, M.C., C.C.D.C., Private Practice, Seattle) and our research consultants (Fred Bookstein, Ph.D., Distinguished Research Scientist; Institute of Gerontology, University of Michigan; Heather Carmichael Olson, Ph.D., FADU; and Sterling Clarren, FAS Diagnostic Clinic, Aldrich Professor of Pediatrics, University of Washington School of Medicine) who worked together to plan and carry out both the research and the conference.

A National Scientific Advisory consisted of Dr. Oakley; Dr. Bookstein; Dr. Clarren; Dr. Lewis Holmes, Chief, Genetics and Teratology Unit, Massachusetts General Hospital; and Dr. Kenneth Warren, Director, Office of Scientific Affairs, National Institute of Alcoholism and Alcohol Abuse.

Preparation of the present book was facilitated by a Review Committee who reviewed and critiqued the manuscripts invited for this volume, which derived from selected papers presented at the conference. This committee included Susan Astley, Ph.D., Heather Carmichael Olson, Ph.D., and Nancy White, then of the Western Washington March of Dimes. Additional reviewers included Fred Bookstein, Ph.D., Sterling Clarren, Ph.D., Paul Sampson, Ph.D., and Kieran O'Malley, M.D. The contributions of this committee in enhancing this volume are gratefully acknowledged.

Acknowledgment is also due to Sharalyn Jackson, dedicated work-study student from Seattle Pacific University who typeset the manuscript, and to the staff at FADU for clerical help and support services.

Naomi Pascal, Associate Director and Editor-in-Chief of the University of Washington Press, was an unfailing source of support and encouragement. Co-Editor Jonathan Kanter, M.A. assumed the bulk of the technical responsibility for editing the manuscripts, sandwiched gracefully between his duties as a Research Assistant and graduate student in the Psychology Department of the University of Washington.

Jonathan and I thank Martin, Zelma, and Laura Kanter, Antoinette Giedzinska, and Daniel Streissguth for their continuing support, confidence, and encouragement.

Finally, we thank the 36 authors who graciously contributed their time and expertise to this volume, including Fred Bookstein, who not only condensed three days of talks into his Rapporteur's Report, but was an active consultant on all stages of the manuscript preparation. This volume is the first to bring together the research and writings of professionals and families working to overcome secondary disabilities in people with Fetal Alcohol Syndrome and Fetal Alcohol Effects. May it not be the last.

All proceeds from the sale of this volume will be used for further applied research on alcohol-related birth defects, through the Fetal Alcohol Research Fund of the University of Washington School of Medicine.

Introduction

Michael Dorris

Eight years ago at the Research Society on Alcoholism meetings in South Carolina I was generally perceived to be the worst kind of pest — a parent with issues. Since then, since *The Broken Cord* was published and then made into a film and translated into languages from Korean to Polish, I have heard from more than four thousand parents much like I was then — desperate and terrified. I have tried to respond to each of them — not with a message of hope for cure, which I cannot offer, but with information and, more importantly, with compassion.

Each parent's tale of their child with Fetal Alcohol Syndrome or Fetal Alcohol Effects is an original script, never before spoken in the light of day, and yet each one of us, almost as if we are compelled to do so, recounts certain basic and similar events, the same disappointments, the same guilts and regrets. All we can wish for from a fellow traveler is understanding, a nod of recognition, a hand on the arm. Empathy — and its more complicated cousin, probably, diagnosis — doesn't solve our problems, or our children's, but it is healing, it is affirming, it is a candle in a long dark corridor.

I am honored to have been asked to introduce this vitally important book, and I do so with the realization that it's not me you're honoring, but Abel, my late, and inspiring son, who should have been nearly thirty years old now, should have been a father, a husband, somebody's wonderful lover, should have contributed to this world by his original acts and not by his sad example. Let me tell you the most remarkable thing about Abel: He lived for 23 years, endured daily loneliness and confusion and hardship and frustration, and in all that time never once did anything that was intentionally cruel or hurtful to another living creature. He was maddening in his inability to learn from experience, to grasp a larger picture, but he was also sweetness distilled. When he visits me in dreams he is always smiling, always forgiving, always advising me not to take everything so seriously. Those graceful qualities made him irresistible, were what shone through the book, were what continue to provoke indignation on his behalf.

If only he had been able to learn how to cross the street in accordance with a green light.

My thoughts here are full of beginnings, pregnant with questions, loaded with stories I want to tell you so that you who are not parents of an alcohol-damaged child will understand what we as a society and as individuals are losing by not solving this preventable scourge.

I was recently in Rangiroa, in the South Pacific and two events there stood out to me as examples I might share.

The first occurred my last night there. A Polynesian family — mother, father, two daughters and a son — invited me for dinner. Afterward we sat on the verandah under a half-full moon and read, passing the book around, the French translation of my young adult book, *Morning Girl*. That two hours was, to me, the epitome of family: sharing, gentle, patient, involved. It was a moment perfectly ordinary to that remote and protected place, where never once in two weeks did I hear a child cry. It was a moment impossible to conceive if one placed within its cast of characters a child or adult afflicted with FAS or FAE. It is *not* a utopian fantasy, I thought as I walked home that night, to imagine that we could, as human beings, learn to be live like that again. It is not crazy to know what to hope for.

The other example from Rangiroa casts me in the role of any of my three adopted alcohol-impaired children. The magazine assignment that sent me to the Tuamotus was to learn to scuba dive in order to write about the adventure. Initially, I pictured myself as Lloyd Bridges in "Sea Hunt." The problem was, all the instruction I received was in French.

"*Tu comprends?*" Manu, my teacher asked solicitously at every stage of the process.

I could sense I was slow, a bit annoying, and so I dutifully answered "*oui,*" even as the truth escalated from "not exactly" to "no way."

Did I actually *comprends,* in the life-and-death sense? Did my children *comprennent* when their learning disabilities specialists or the police or their parole officers explained to them the basic operating instructions for survival in a world in which they had no bearings? Did they *comprennent* the meaning of limits, the necessity of thought before action?

No. Like me, they depended at first on one-on-one guidance, which worked for a little while. And when that stopped, when they or I were expected to have learned the rules, mastered the game, be independent and be left solo, did we truly know what to do?

No, again. I was actually swept out to sea in a strong undercurrent that, though I was later assured it had been explained to me, was one of those features that I didn't sufficiently comprehend. I was barely saved. My older children similarly were swept into the chaos of a demanding society — and they were lost. When you don't understand how things work, your chances for success are slim.

Another beginning. The other day I was in a toy store in Pioneer Square in Seattle with my three healthy, normal, younger daughters. The first thing that caught my eye was a novelty toy called "The Incredible Brain." There it was, this little plastic fist of potential — and the directions seemed so simple.

How To Make Your Brain Grow!

Fill a large container (jar, bottle, sink or tub) with water. Place your new brain in the container. Stand back! Just kidding. Actually, it takes up to 48 hours for your brain to reach it's full growing potential. Show it to your friends, they'll be amazed!

But what if one screwed up, put the new brain into ethanol rather than water and it didn't grow. Instead, its convolutions smoothed out, stayed small, did not fill its cranial container. The moral is: It's not enough to follow the directions. You have to employ the right ingredients to start with.

FAS is the last thing on earth I ever wanted to be "expert" on. We fall into our fates, or leap unknowingly into them, and then we try to figure them out as best we can. Albert Camus once said that it was the writer's job to speak for those without a voice. Perhaps the job of a parent of a child with FAS or FAE is purely to rage and howl for his children — or for those who entrust to him or her their anonymous tragedies. For seven years I have opened nearly every day the letters of strangers, letters demanding to be contradicted. Letters about cosmic unfairness, waste, broken marriages, crime, far reaching consequences, good intentions turned into bitter cynicism. Their authors call out to you today through me. "If you can't help our children," they cry, "make sure this never happens again. Our hands are full, so we depend on you, those not directly involved. *Do* the impossible." I join their plea: *end* this cycle of woe. Let the beginning of its eradication start here, today. A quarter of a century ago scholars at the University of Washington first had the imagination to identify the culprit, first made the logical leap, put two and two together and came up with four: Whatever goes into the mother's body becomes the consuming environment for the fetus she harbors.

What have I learned from these chronicles? Certainly, that ordinary people can rise to courage and perseverance, can remain loyal to their ideals. But also, in chorus, they alert me to the relatively small effect of environment on changing the inevitable. One can surely make a bad condition worse by abuse or neglect or denial or failure to obtain an early explanatory diagnosis, but one can't create *ex post facto* what was inhibited from natural development. Whether my letters come from Malaysia or Miami, from India or Indiana, there is a chilling uniformity in the appearance of defining symptoms. 'Predestination' is too mild a word to describe the steady march from "small, cute and *so* affectionate," to an individual's struggle to learn how to tell time, to retain the multiplication tables, to not shoplift. There is a typical FAS/FAE trajectory — *de*jectory is probably the better term — with which parents and professionals responsible for these brain- and body-damaged people are all too familiar: Things almost always get worse with the passage of time.

As those of us in the field know well, once involved it's hard to quit. FAS engages our emotions, our sense that justice has been violated, our impulse to put out the fire before the forest is ablaze. It regularly challenges our politics because its hypothetical solutions sometimes go against the grain of our allegiance to universal and absolute human rights. It sets up profoundly agonizing conflicts of interest that go to the core of our ethical beings: What takes precedence, the right of a woman to decide what to ingest into her own body or the right to wholeness of the child she has elected to carry to term? Do protocols protecting client or community confidentiality or privacy *always* supersede the public need for every scrap of useful data, even if it's only evidence of the magnitude and scope of the problem? In matters of life and death, some armchair principles seem less than immutable, some rules may need to be humanely bent. One thing is sure: Bureaucracies positively impede progress and obscure the truth.

But who's going to blow *that* whistle and never receive another dime of funding, plus risk the censure of the purists, the disapprobation of those lucky enough not to have to face the issues head-on, daily, hourly? Who's going to tell the hard truths: We need a new Australia, where many victims of the so-called "gin epidemic" two hundred years ago were exiled and, deprived of alcohol, bore healthy offspring? We may well need to create a set of mandatory farms or protected rural living environments which stress repetitive tasks and are permanently tuned in to the cartoon channel. We need oversight for those who can't or don't foresee enough to protect themselves.

In reviewing reports of FAS-related projects around the country sponsored by the Centers for Disease Control, I was struck by a fact that is rarely mentioned — perhaps because it is so overwhelming in its implications. The vast majority of people afflicted with FAS or FAE in this world are not children, but adults. Unless some of them become — as often they do — mothers of a next generation of FAS-impaired infants, they rarely get diagnosed or counted. In my experience, their life-long brain and motor damage is not even tentatively identified until a court sentencing hearing in which a savvy public defender of a seemingly remorseless criminal gets the bright idea of an FAE-mitigating strategy.

It's a facile but short-sighted policy to act as though FAS is an issue confined to children under twelve years old, or to women. There is no logical cutoff point in the population because innate disability — physical or mental — interacts with social environments and shifting expectations in different ways throughout a person's lifetime. Behaviors that are tolerable though worrisome at eleven become unacceptable and criminal at fifteen, prosecutable at eighteen, thuggish at forty. Unless we are willing to accept a Brave New World scenario with a constantly increasing percentage of middle-aged "gammas" — some of them dangerous to themselves and others, all of them permanently confused and requiring the enactment of generalized laws that are more and more restrictive (for all of us) to replace the normal cultural ability to interact with common assumptions, to learn from example or experience — we must redefine FAS as an issue that cuts in varying but real ways across every sector and age group of the population, both genders, all social and economic demographics.

I can't demonstrate this to you with color transparencies, statistical analyses or cautious peer-reviewed conclusions. I am in many respects today what I was eight years ago — an implacable, desperate parent with issues, knocking, pounding on the door. One of my children is dead, one has been diagnosed by a court-ordered psychiatrist as homicidal, violent and obsessive, the last is selling crank — and herself — on the streets of a western city, when she isn't practicing her own wacky brand of Satanism. This is in spite of hundreds of thousands of dollars expended on "special" schools, counseling, rehabilitation, in spite of Covenant House, Boys Town and Casey Family Services, in spite of prison and boot camp and the Job Corps. In spite of the fact that though they will always be my children and hence I will always love them as such I must, for the safety of myself and my family, strictly maintain a physical and emotional distance from them — possibly forever.

Let me conclude with more stories to illustrate how far we have yet to go.

For a while I believed my wife and I had done our little part — and Abel his big one — with *The Broken Cord*. I thought it had reached a lot of people, a critical mass, and had made some dent of difference. I thought I could go back to doing what I love to do: writing fiction.

It's not that easy. I've reluctantly embarked on a new book titled *Matter of Conscience* about that ephemeral collection of otherwise inexplicable symptoms heretofore known as Fetal Alcohol Effects. I don't look forward to doing it; I thought I was done.

I made the decision to do this book, however, because of three incidents of the past year that demonstrated to me in how much trouble we as a society still find ourselves.

The first two involve smart, highly educated, powerful professional women whom I met in New York last spring. One had given birth to a son two years before and told me how her Park Avenue obstetrician greeted her with a martini at her standing Friday 5:15 appointment — to calm her down after a stressful work week. Sometimes the exam concluded with a second round. She had no idea he was potentially feeding her baby poison.

The second woman, equally impressive in her career, had recently been a week late in delivering her baby. *Her* Park Avenue obstetrician/gynecologist advised, "Oh, relax and take the Italian solution": In other words, go home, drink a *bottle* of Chianti, and have great sex.

"I did it for four nights," she confided to me, "but after all I still had to be induced."

Four bottles of Chianti, one after another, during one of the most critical periods of fetal brain development. Doctor's orders. Paid for, no doubt, by a corporate HMO.

Finally, I knew I had to do this book when I received a call from an Indian Health hospital in the Pacific Northwest. The nurse had read *The Broken Cord* some years ago, and just hours before she had delivered from my 38-year-old unmarried alcoholic cousin a full FAS-diagnosed neonate.

"I thought you'd like to know," this anonymous voiced woman told me over the phone. "She named him after you. Michael Dorris."

I don't just owe my continuing efforts to faceless infants and adults, I owe it to my namesake, I owe it to my children, I owe it to me.

Let me end by offering the first paragraph of what I hope will become *Matter of Conscience*, to be published in the fall of 1998.

I am society, and my life is in threat. I believed I could alter fate. I tried and failed, in process with lapses of patience and with anger, and ultimately because I had no choice but not to give up. I intended nothing but good, though I expected to be rewarded with gratitude and love, and I wound up the center of a target. I imagined myself powerful, but now I awake every night consumed by dread, by fear. I was foolhardy, a fool. I was driven temporarily mad and may never fully recover enough to completely recall the person I think I used to be. I tried to save three lives: Maybe I didn't try hard enough. Maybe they were unstable. One is gone. One is lost. One is a danger to anyone within his line of sight. I wish I had reconciled earlier to the impossibility of my goal. I wish the conclusion that faces me was avoidable. I wish I could return to do it again, so as perhaps not to do it again, at least not as blindly as I did it the first time. I want my life back. I want my peaceful sleep. I want to fear once again only those natural human fears. I wish my adopted children to achieve amnesia or, better, to remember the entirety of their lives with me. I want them to be well. I want justice. I want reasonable hope for a future untainted by preventable tragedy. I want my and my children's experience to spare just one life, for all of the sorrow to balance a single redemption. I want my children's lives to have mattered.

Fetal Alcohol Syndrome can be eliminated, but it's a slow and painstaking process. Progress moves slowly, one rescued human life at a time.

The Challenge of Fetal Alcohol Syndrome

Overcoming Secondary Disabilities

Neurobehavioral and Neuroanatomical Effects of Heavy Prenatal Exposure to Alcohol

Sarah N. Mattson and Edward P. Riley

Introduction

It has now been over 20 years since the identification of Fetal Alcohol Syndrome (FAS) and our knowledge about the effects of prenatal alcohol exposure has increased tremendously. We have gone from a simple description of the physical features related to heavy alcohol exposure to identifying potential mechanisms of alcohol's teratogenicity. Similarly, we have moved from identifying facial features associated with the syndrome to trying to understand the underlying causes for alcohol's effect on the developing facies. We certainly have much more to accomplish, however, and as in the past, these accomplishments will be based upon both animal and human studies (Driscoll, Streissguth, & Riley, 1990).

Although there has been much discussion about the diagnosis of FAS during the last two decades, the diagnosis of FAS still remains much the same as originally proposed by Jones and Smith (1973). The diagnosis is based on a triad of features: (1) pre- and/or postnatal growth deficiency; (2) a distinct pattern of craniofacial malformations; and (3) central nervous system (CNS) dysfunction. The growth deficits noted in the neonatal period (Jones & Smith, 1973) often continue through adolescence and adulthood (Streissguth, Aase et al., 1991). The pattern of facial malformations includes short palpebral fissures, a long smooth philtrum, a thin vermilion border, and flat midface (Jones & Smith, 1973). The CNS dysfunction is variable and can present as microcephaly, structural brain anomalies, and various neurological or behavioral signs such as gait problems, hyperactivity, attention deficits, learning disabilities, or mental retardation (Stratton, Howe, & Battaglia, 1996).

Soon after FAS was originally identified, it became obvious that not all children exposed to large amounts of alcohol prenatally had

This paper was supported by the National Institute on Alcohol Abuse and Alcoholism grant # AA10417.

all of the diagnostic criteria necessary to warrant a diagnosis of FAS. Estimates of the number of diagnosable FAS cases among heavily drinking women have been placed at between 10 and 40 percent (Jones & Smith, 1975). Also, it became obvious that although these children had escaped the facial dysmorphology that is required for the FAS diagnosis, they were still at risk for serious behavioral and cognitive problems. There have been many labels proposed to identify these children, including Fetal Alcohol Effects (FAE), Alcohol Related Birth Defects (ARBD), and the most recent Alcohol Related Neurodevelopmental Disorder (ARND) (Stratton, Howe, & Battaglia, 1996). In our work we have referred to these individuals as Prenatal Exposure to Alcohol (PEA) because they have confirmed histories of prenatal alcohol exposure, but lack the features of the Fetal Alcohol Syndrome. In fact, in our cases they typically have few if any of the defining physical characteristics of FAS. One of the most intriguing and important questions facing researchers who study the effects of prenatal alcohol exposure is how to better identify these children and discover the features that may in some way distinguish them from children showing similar behavioral and cognitive features attributable to another developmental disability.

The behavioral and cognitive effects of prenatal alcohol are among the most devastating consequences of such exposure and characterization of these effects might increase our understanding of how alcohol affects the developing brain. The purpose of this review is to overview the findings of several domains of cognitive functioning in children exposed prenatally to alcohol with special attention on our recent work in this area. A discussion of alterations in brain structures resulting from such exposure will also be presented, again with an emphasis on our recent imaging work.

The Effects of Prenatal Alcohol Exposure on Intelligence

Although the diagnosis of FAS does not require mental retardation, general intellectual functioning is often compromised. In fact, FAS is thought to be the leading known cause of mental retardation in the Western world (Abel & Sokol, 1987). A recent survey of the FAS case reports between 1973 and 1996 in which an exact IQ estimate was provided, found a mean IQ of 65.73 (SD = 20.2) with a range of 20 to 120 (Mattson & Riley, 1996). A similar review (Mattson & Riley, 1996) of larger retrospective studies of groups of children with FAS reported between 1974 and 1996 (Majewski, 1978; 1978; Olegård et al., 1979; Streissguth, Herman, & Smith, 1978; Streissguth & Rohsenow, 1974) resulted in a mean IQ of 72.26 (range

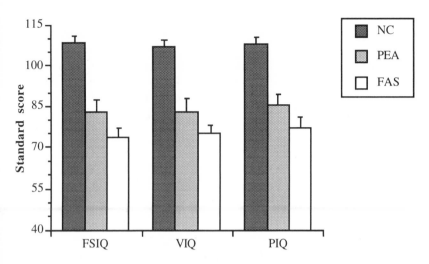

Figure 1. IQ scores of children with FAS and PEA, and normal controls (NC). FSIQ, full scale IQ; VIQ, verbal IQ; PIQ, performance IQ. (From Mattson, Riley, Gramling, Delis, & Jones, in press-b.)

of means, 47.4 to 98.2). Thus, it appears that the IQ of the average person with FAS falls in the borderline range of mental retardation, although there is a substantial amount of variation resulting in a wide range of IQ scores.

Importantly, even in the absence of the specific facial malformations, and thus the absence of the diagnosis of FAS, cognitive deficits, including mental retardation, can still be present. For example, we (Mattson, Riley, Gramling, Delis, & Jones, in press-a) recently evaluated the overall level of intellectual functioning in children with FAS and PEA using the age appropriate Wechsler Intelligence Test (Wechsler, 1989; 1974). Recall that children with PEA have confirmed histories of heavy prenatal exposure to alcohol but have few, if any, of the physical anomalies required for a diagnosis of FAS. The results from these IQ assessments are presented in Figure 1.

The children with FAS have IQ scores in the low-to-mid 70s which is consistent with previous reports. What is interesting and perhaps important about these data is that the PEA children are scoring in the low 80s. These are children with few if any of the stigmata associated with FAS, yet they are scoring in the low-average range. Although in this particular study the differences between the FAS and PEA groups were not significant, it does appear that children with FAS are more affected than are those that we refer to as PEA. This relationship, which is similar to a "dose-response relationship," with diagnostic group as the defining factor, is illustrated in the figure. These data are similar to those previously reported by Streissguth, Aase, and colleagues (1991). It should also be mentioned that exposure to as little as one ounce of alcohol per day has been associated with IQ decrements of six to seven points (Streissguth, Barr, & Sampson, 1990).

Language

In several case reports of children with FAS, speech and language disturbances have been mentioned. Abel (1990) noted about 10% of the cases surveyed reported speech delays or impediments. Additionally, there have been reports of both receptive (Shaywitz, Caparulo, & Hodgson, 1981) and expressive (Tenbrinck & Buchin, 1975) deficits. Russell, Czarnecki, Cowan, McPherson, and Mudar (1991) reported that receptive language functioning was related to indications of maternal problem drinking. Similarly, Streissguth, Barr, Olson, and colleagues (1994) found a relationship between maternal alcohol intake and performance on the Word Attack test which assesses knowledge of pronunciation rules.

In a recent study (Mattson, Riley, Delis, Stern, & Jones, in press-a), we assessed language functioning. Children with FAS and PEA were administered the Peabody Picture Vocabulary Test-Revised (PPVT-R; Dunn & Dunn, 1981) and the Boston Naming Test (BNT; Kaplan, Goodglass, & Weintraub, 1983), which address word comprehension and naming ability, respectively. Similar to the findings with overall IQ scores (Mattson, Riley, Gramling, Delis, & Jones, in press-b), the FAS and PEA children were impaired to a similar degree when compared to controls although the children with FAS appeared to be slightly more impaired than were the children with PEA (Mattson, Riley, Gramling, Delis, & Jones, in press-a).

Visuospatial Functioning

Although rats exposed to alcohol prenatally are known to have deficits on tasks involving spatial abilities (Gianoulakis, 1990; Kelly, Goodlett, Hulsether, & West, 1988; Reyes, Wolfe, & Savage, 1989), very little work has been done in this domain with children with FAS. Streissguth, Sampson, and colleagues (1994) reported deficits in spatial learning on the stepping stone maze in 14-year-old children. This test measures short-term recall of complex spatial patterns. Additionally, at 7.5 years of age, a visuoconstructional task was one of the most sensitive measures of alcohol's teratogenesis (Streissguth,

Bookstein, Sampson, & Barr, 1989). Recently, Uecker and Nadel (1996) reported that children with FAS or FAE were significantly impaired in delayed, but not immediate, recall for information involving spatial location. These same children also were able to recall a series of objects but not their spatial locations.

We recently documented an interesting visuospatial deficit in a group of alcohol-exposed children (Mattson, Gramling, Delis, Jones & Riley, 1996). By asking children to recall hierarchical visual stimuli, we found differential deficits in the processing of global vs. local visual features. The Global-Local Test assesses hierarchical visual processing and has been used to distinguish between patients with right and left hemisphere focal brain damage (Delis, Keifner, & Fridlund, 1988), as well as between children with different types of developmental disorders (Bihrle, Bellugi, Delis, & Marks, 1989). Using this test, we determined that alcohol-exposed children focus on the global aspects of visual stimuli at the expense of the local details when asked to recall a hierarchical stimulus consisting of large ("global") and small ("local") components. Of equal interest was the fact that the dissociation of global and local features was also present when the memory component was removed by having the child copy the hierarchical stimulus. Thus, even with the image in full view, the alcohol-exposed children had difficulty copying the local aspects of the figure. These deficits were not due to visual problems, since they occurred only when hierarchical stimuli were presented and not when single level stimuli were used, regardless of their size.

Similar work in other groups of children with developmental disorders suggests that this sort of deficit in local processing clusters with relative strengths in the nonverbal domain of cognition. For example, children with Down syndrome, who typically have greater nonverbal than verbal abilities, showed similar deficits to those of FAS children while children with Williams syndrome, which is characterized by a high degree of verbal fluency, showed the opposite pattern (Bihrle, Bellugi, Delis, & Marks, 1989). Similarly, in a study of patients with Alzheimer's disease, those who showed relative sparing of nonverbal abilities also showed global preference while those with better verbal abilities were more likely to do better on the local aspects of this task (Delis, Massman et al., 1992). Finally, in developmentally normal adults with acquired brain damaged, a deficit in local processing is present in patients with left hemisphere lesions (Delis, Kiefner, & Fridlund, 1988).

Children with FAS, PEA, and normal controls were also evaluated using Beery's Developmental Test of Visual-Motor Integration (VMI), a drawing test in which the child has to copy increasingly difficult line drawings (Beery, 1989). On this measure, as in the overall IQ and language measures, alcohol-exposed children performed more poorly than did matched controls, with little difference between the FAS and PEA children. In terms of standardized scores, the normal controls had a mean of 95.2 compared to 80.3 and 83.5 for the FAS and PEA groups, respectively (Mattson, Riley, Gramling, Delis, & Jones, in press-a).

Verbal Learning and Memory

It also appears that verbal memory is affected by prenatal alcohol exposure. For example, deficits have been noted in story memory (Streissguth, Bookstein, Sampson, & Barr, 1989) and working memory (Kodituwakku, Handmaker, Cutler, Weathersby, & Handmaker, 1995). Recently, we (Mattson, Riley, Delis, Stern, & Jones, 1996) assessed 20 children with FAS and matched controls using the California Verbal Learning Test–Children's Version (CVLT-C; Delis, Kramer, Kaplan, & Ober, 1994), a list-learning task that assesses various aspects of verbal learning and memory. The CVLT-C consists of five learning trials, in each of which a 15-word list is presented. Although the child is not told, this list can be clustered into three semantic categories: fruit, toys, and clothes. After the five immediate recall trials, a second, distracter list is presented. Next, the child is asked to recall the words on the initial list and is then provided with the semantic categories to aid his or her recall. Following a 20-minute delay, this free and cued recall procedure is repeated. In this way both short and long delay, free and cued recall measures are obtained. Finally, a 45-word yes/no recognition test is given. When compared to age-matched control children, the children with FAS had difficulty learning and recalling the words after short and long delays. That is, they recalled fewer words on all the initial learning trials as well as on the short and long delay recall trials. Their pattern of recall suggested deficits in encoding verbal material, although the learning strategies they used were similar to controls and their retention of learned material was relatively intact. Interestingly, in recalling the words, these children made an increased number of intrusions, perseverations, and false positive errors. These types of errors are consistent with a response inhibition deficit which has previously been reported in alcohol-exposed children and animals (Driscoll, Streissguth, & Riley, 1990).

Motor Abilities

Although there are exceptions (Chandler, Richardson, Gallagher, & Day, 1996; Forrest, Florey, Taylor, McPherson, & Young, 1991;

Fried, O'Connell, & Watkinson, 1992; Fried & Watkinson, 1990), most studies of motor development and motor skills suggest impairment due to prenatal alcohol exposure, perhaps implicating some cerebellar dysfunction. Animal studies have revealed that prenatal and neonatal alcohol exposure leads to deficits in behaviors linked to the cerebellum (Goodlett, Thomas, & West, 1991). In humans, there have been several reports of motor dysfunction following heavy prenatal alcohol exposure. Delayed motor development and fine-motor dysfunction were noted in the first descriptions of children with FAS (Jones, Smith, Ulleland, & Streissguth, 1973). Soon after, an additional report noted a "non-specific dyscoordinated motor pattern," hemiplegia, ataxia, and an increase in cerebral palsy in children of alcohol-abusing women (Olegård et al., 1979). Similarly, Marcus (1987) noted axial ataxia and kinetic tremor in children with FAS. Delayed motor development has been linked to prenatal alcohol exposure in infants and children (Autti-Rämö & Granström, 1991; Jacobson et al., 1993; Streissguth, Barr, Martin, & Herman, 1980) and fine and gross motor dysfunction was noted in children of alcoholic mothers (Kyllerman et al., 1985) and social drinkers (Barr, Streissguth, Darby, & Sampson, 1990). Finally, FAS has been associated with decrements in motor speed and precision, finger tapping speed, and grip strength (Conry, 1990; Janzen, Nanson, & Block, 1995; Mattson, Riley, Gramling, Delis, & Jones, in press-a).

Attention

Deficits in attention have long been associated with prenatal alcohol exposure. The earliest studies noted an increased "non-alert state" in infants who were exposed to alcohol prenatally. These infants spent more time with eyes open, but not attending (Landesman-Dwyer, Keller, & Streissguth, 1978). These alcohol-related attentional deficits appear to continue through childhood and may be similar to those seen in children with attention deficit disorder (ADD) (Nanson & Hiscock, 1990). Children with FAS/FAE or ADD both displayed deficits in investing, organizing, and maintaining attention as well as an increase in impulsive responding. Similarly, adolescents and adults with FAS demonstrated deficits in tasks involved in focusing, encoding, and shifting attention (Olson, Feldman, Streissguth, & Gonzalez, 1992). However, in another study, children with FAS/FAE performed similarly to controls and better than children with ADD on tests of reaction time and vigilance (Coles et al., 1997).

Attentional deficits have also been related to prenatal alcohol exposure in children without FAS. Four-year-old children of "social drinkers" were observed to have poorer attention spans than control children when parity, maternal smoking, home environment, and sex of child were used as covariates (Landesman-Dwyer, Ragozin, & Little, 1981). Streissguth and colleagues have noted alcohol-related attentional deficits at ages four (Streissguth et al., 1984), seven (Streissguth, Barr et al., 1986), eleven (Olson, Sampson, Barr, Streissguth, & Bookstein, 1992), and fourteen (Streissguth, Barr, Sampson et al., 1994; Streissguth, Sampson et al., 1994). Streissguth's findings were supported by Brown and colleagues (1991) who reported deficits in the ability to sustain attention following alcohol exposure throughout pregnancy.

Neuroanatomical Features of FAS and PEA

Although it is clear that alcohol is a physical and behavioral terat-ogen, its teratogenic effects on the developing brain have often been difficult to quantify. Certainly, the multitude of behavioral and cognitive studies should allow an inference about the state of the brain, but specific details about structural brain damage in humans are limited. There is no question that prenatal exposure to high levels of alcohol affects the developing brain, however, whether this expo-sure results in a specific pattern of brain damage is still questioned. This section addresses the brain anomalies that have been reported following prenatal alcohol exposure, from the early autopsy studies to the more recent imaging studies.

In the first report of Jones and Smith (1973), the authors described an infant with FAS who died shortly after birth. An autopsy of this child revealed extensive brain damage which included microcephaly, migration anomalies, callosal dysgenesis, and a "massive" neuroglial, leptomeningeal heterotopia covering the left hemisphere. Soon after this report, Clarren (1977) described a second infant, born to a binge drinker, who died at 10 days of age. This autopsy revealed severe hydrocephalus, abnormal neuronal migration, and size reductions of the corpus callosum and cerebellum. Since then, prenatal alcohol exposure has also been linked to brainstem and cerebellar anomalies, agenesis of the corpus callosum and anterior commissure, migration errors, absent olfactory bulbs, hydrocephalus, meningomyelocele, and porencephaly (Clarren, 1986; Clarren, Alvord, Sumi, Streissguth, & Smith, 1978; Goldstein & Arulanantham, 1978; Peiffer, Majewski, Fischbach, Bierich, & Volk, 1979; Wisniewski, Dambska, Sher, & Qazi, 1983). Currently, reports of 25 autopsies appear in the litera-ture. A review of these cases can be found elsewhere (Mattson & Riley, in press). Although some (Clarren, 1986; Peiffer, Majewski,

Fischbach, Bierich, & Volk, 1979) believe that the nature of the brain damage resulting from prenatal alcohol exposure is extremely variable, more recent advances in brain imaging technology which allow a more systematic measure of alcohol's teratogenicity have provided data to the contrary. The following is a brief summary of the results of our recent Magnetic Resonance Imaging (MRI) studies of children with FAS and PEA.

Case Reports

Initially we (Mattson et al., 1994; Mattson et al., 1992) analyzed the MRIs of four children exposed to alcohol prenatally and fully processed the images to obtain the following volumetric measures: overall cerebral vault, cerebellar vault, basal ganglia, and diencephalon. Of these four children, two met the traditional criteria for FAS while the other two were PEA children. All four children had decreased volumes of the cerebral and cerebellar vaults. In addition, both the FAS and PEA children had decreases in the volume of the basal ganglia, even when overall brain size was accounted for by using proportion of volume of the basal ganglia to overall brain volume. Alternatively, only the children with the characteristics of FAS displayed disproportionate reductions in the diencephalon.

Corpus Callosum

The corpus callosum is a large fiber tract that connects the two hemispheres of the brain. Because of earlier case reports of agenesis of the corpus callosum and callosal thinning, we evaluated the size of this structure in children with histories of significant prenatal alcohol exposure, many of whom met the criteria for FAS (Riley et al., 1995). Using MRI images of the mid-sagittal section and a computer-assisted digitizing system, the area of the corpus callosum was measured. In addition to measuring the overall area, the corpus callosum was divided into five equiangular regions and each of these five regions was measured. When compared to a group of normal control children, the alcohol-exposed children had significantly smaller overall corpus callosum areas, as well as smaller areas for four of the five callosal regions. Furthermore, when overall brain size was accounted for, reductions were found in three of the five callosal regions. These findings are illustrated in Figure 2. Similar results have been reported in children with attention deficit hyperactivity disorder (Hynd et al., 1991) which is an extremely interesting finding given the high prevalence of attention deficits in children with FAS.

Also of note is the finding of three cases of agenesis of the corpus callosum in our sample. Although not all children in our larger

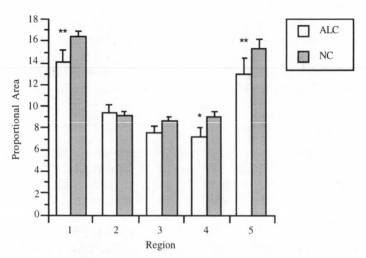

Figure 2. Mean proportional area of five regions of the corpus callosum in alcohol-exposed children (ALC) and normal controls (NC). *p<0.05, **p<0.01 (From Riley et al., 1995.)

sample have received MRI scans, the present incidence of agenesis of the corpus callosum in this sample is 3/44 or 6.8%. This is considerably higher than the rate of 0.3% in the general population and even the rate of 2.3% in developmentally disabled populations (Jeret, Serur, Wisniewski, & Lubin, 1987; Jeret, Serur, Wisniewski, & Fisch, 1986).

Cerebellar Vermis

We recently reviewed the MRIs of children and young adults exposed to alcohol prenatally and assessed the area of the cerebellar vermis (Sowell et al., 1996). Using the mid-sagittal section, three vermal regions were defined: anterior vermis (vermal lobules I-V), posterior vermis (vermal lobules VI-VII), and the remaining vermal region (vermal lobules VIII-X). When compared to age-matched normal controls, the area of the anterior vermal region was smaller in the alcohol-exposed subjects, although the posterior region and remaining vermal regions of both groups were similar in size. These data are illustrated in Figure 3.

Basal Ganglia

As mentioned previously, the volume of the basal ganglia was found to be reduced in the first four MRI evaluations done. We have

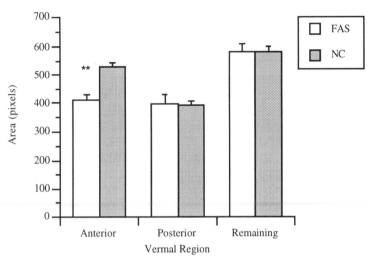

Figure 3. Area of three regions of the cerebellar vermis in children with FAS and normal controls (NC). ** $p<0.01$ (From Mattson & Riley, in press.)

examined six additional MRIs using a newly revised MRI protocol. The results are consistent with our previous report and indicate that the basal ganglia are reduced in volume in children exposed to alcohol prenatally. Further, it appears that within the basal ganglia, the caudate nucleus but not the lenticular nuclei is reduced (Mattson, Riley, Sowell et al., 1996). The functional ramifications of these reductions in the basal ganglia are currently under study.

Summary

In summary, prenatal alcohol exposure is associated with a wide range of neuropsychological and neuroanatomical abnormalities. These effects appear to be similar in children with FAS and those who were exposed to high levels of alcohol but who do not have the characteristics required for the diagnosis of FAS. This emphasizes the pervasive nature of alcohol's teratogenicity and the importance of identifying children who are at risk due to prenatal alcohol exposure, even if they do not meet the criteria for FAS. Specifically, alcohol-exposed children, with and without FAS, displayed deficits in verbal learning, language, some aspects of visuospatial ability, as well as overall intellectual ability. Neuroanatomically, prenatal alcohol exposure has been linked to reductions in the corpus callosum, basal ganglia and portions of the cerebellar vermis, as well as overall cerebrum and cerebellar volume.

Although prenatal alcohol exposure appears to have pervasive and often devastating consequences, the data presented herein emphasize that a specific pattern of results may still be found in individuals with FAS and PEA. For example, learning deficits along with relatively spared retention were found on the CVLT-C. Similarly, with MRI studies, reductions in the caudate nucleus but not the lenticular nuclei were found in children with FAS. Future research in both animals and humans should continue to focus on specific aspects of prenatal alcohol exposure so that the pattern of structural and functional outcomes (both spared and impaired) can be more clearly defined. It is only with this degree of detail that specific strategies for remediation can be designed.

Children of Alcoholic Mothers: Results from Göteborg, Sweden

Marita Aronson

Introduction

The effects of alcohol on the developing fetus have been well recognized for about 25 years. The fetal toxicity of alcohol has been confirmed by several groups around the world (Lemoine, Harrousseau, Borteyru, & Mennet, 1968; Jones & Smith, 1975; Bierich, Majewski, & Michaelis, 1975; Olegård et al., 1979). In the 1970's and 1980's our research group in Göteborg reported on the consequences of alcohol on the growing fetus and child (Olegård et al., 1979; Aronson, 1984; Aronson & Olegård, 1987; Aronson, Kyllerman, Sabel, Sandin, & Olegård, 1985; Kyllerman et al., 1985; Streissguth, Clarren, & Jones, 1985). Follow-up studies have been few, partly because this field of research is new, and partly because there have been problems tracing the examination groups for follow-up. Studies on the intermediate and long-term outcome of children born to alcoholic parents recently have been reported from the United States, France, and Germany (Streissguth, Clarren, & Jones, 1985; Streissguth, Aase et al., 1991; Lemoine & Lemoine, 1992; Steinhausen, 1995). Streissguth's study demonstrated the continuing impact of prenatal alcohol exposure on attention, reaction time, intelligence, memory, learning (particularly in the field of arithmetic), and other neuropsychological functions (Streissguth, Clarren, & Jones, 1985; Streissguth, Aase et al., 1991). Steinhausen (1995) indicated the persistence of hyperkinesis, sleep disorders and stereotypies in adolescence. Lemoine's follow-up study of 105 adult patients with Fetal Alcohol Syndrome suggested that mental retardation, other learning disabilities, behavior problems and "instability" may be common outcomes (Lemoine & Lemoine, 1992).

Outcomes of the Göteborg Studies of Children of Alcoholic Mothers

Our research group has previously published three studies of children exposed to alcohol in utero. In a *retrospective* study (Olegård et al., 1979; Aronson, 1984; Aronson & Olegård, 1987), 99 children, between the ages of 2.5 and 30, of 30 alcoholic mothers were observed. Fifty percent had delayed development and a majority required special education or placement in schools for handicapped children. Fifty percent had specific neuropsychological deficits, making it more difficult for them to make good use of their intellectual resources. Four percent of the children suffered from mild cerebral paresis.

In a *matched comparison group* study (Aronson, Kyllerman, Sabel, Sandin, & Olegård, 1985; Kyllerman et al., 1985), 21 of the 99 children (average age, 5.5 years) were compared to a comparison group, matched for sex, age, height, birth weight and social circumstances. The comparison group showed normal development. Children of alcoholic mothers, on the other hand, demonstrated no significant gain in growth rate, and motor and psychological development levels were considerably below those of the comparison group. We found a high rate of indices of brain dysfunction (including mental retardation) even among those children who had been placed in foster homes at an early age.

In a *prospective* study (Aronson, 1984; Aronson & Olegård, 1987), 26 children (16 boys, 10 girls) and their alcoholic mothers were followed through the pre-school years and given medical and psychological examinations. Mothers with alcohol abuse during pregnancy were questioned with a structured interview at the first visit to the maternal clinic. Two specially trained nurses offered a comprehensive support program for the mothers. The mothers' alcohol consumption was monitored during pregnancy. Of the 26 children, 11 had Fetal Alcohol Syndrome (FAS), 9 had Fetal Alcohol Effects (FAE), and 6 had no physical abnormalities or mental retardation.

The children were divided into four groups according to the amount of alcohol consumption of their mothers during pregnancy:

Group 1: Children whose mothers ended their alcohol abuse at 5 to 12 weeks of gestation (2 boys, 3 girls);

Group 2: Children whose mothers ended consumption at 20 to 25 weeks gestation (6 boys, 1 girl);

Group 3: Children whose mothers consumed alcohol throughout pregnancy (5 boys, 4 girls);

Group 4: Children whose mothers *abused* alcohol (20 centiliters or more of hard liquor per day) throughout the pregnancy but were not discovered as alcoholics and were not in the help program (3 boys, 3 girls).

Group 1 children had normal growth and mental development during pre-school years. Conversely, group 3 and group 4 children had low birth weight and were delayed in their mental development. Group 4 children were discovered after birth and showed signs of FAS. The average age of the mothers at the time of delivery was 21.8 years (range, 19.6 to 24.3) for group 1, 29.9 years (range, 24.9 to 33.1) for group 2, 28.5 years (range, 24.3 to 39.2) for group 3 and 29.2 years (range, 21.6 to 33.1) for group 4.

A Follow-up of the Prospective Study

The 26 children were contacted again in 1990 and 1991, when their ages ranged from 11.5 to 14 years. Two of the children had moved abroad and could not be examined. For two of the remaining 24 children, information could only be obtained from school records. The remaining 22 individuals were clinically and neuropsychologically examined. (A WISC IQ score was available for one additional girl.) Twenty of these were examined by a psychologist blind to the group status and diagnosis.

The foster or biological parents were interviewed in detail about the child's development and behavior for about 60 minutes. The classroom teacher was interviewed about the child's behavior and achievement in the school for about 30 minutes. The child was tested on the test battery and was observed with regard to attention level, distractibility, activity level, social interaction, communication, and overall behavior (including compulsive behaviors, rituals, tics, and stereotypes). The test battery included the WISC-R (Wechsler Intelligence Scale for Children, 1980), the Bender (Koppitz, 1971), the Raven test (Raven, Court, & Raven, 1986; and Raven, Court, & Raven, 1988), and the Draw-A-Man test.

Results

Neuropsychological findings. Figure 1 presents the WISC-R IQ scores by exposure groups. Four children were mildly mentally retarded and had tested IQ scores in the range of 51 to 72. Two of these had neonatally diagnosed FAS (one from group 4 — the severe abuse group, and one from group 2 — the moderate abuse group). The remaining 19 children for whom WISC results were available had IQ scores of 73 or higher, and their mean IQ was 91 (standard deviation 10.3).

Children in group 3 and 4 — the severe abuse groups — had the lowest scores. The five children in group 4, who had been diagnosed

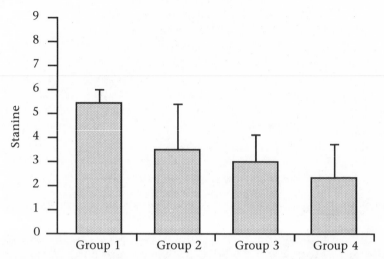

Figure 1. Mean WISC-R IQ scores (+ 1 s.d.) of children in different prenatal exposure groups. Data expressed in stanines — standardized scores with a mean of 5 and a standard deviation of 2. (A stanine of 5 is equivalent to an IQ of 100; a stanine of 3 is equivalent to an IQ of 85.)

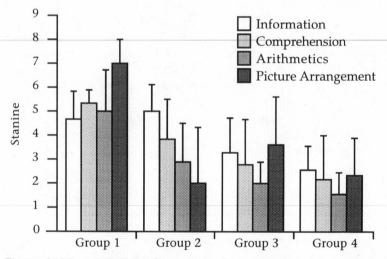

Figure 2. Mean WISC-R subtest scores for comprehension, arithmetic, and picture arrangement for children in different prenatal exposure groups.

with FAS at birth, showed pronounced difficulties on the following subtests: comprehension, arithmetic, picture arrangement, and

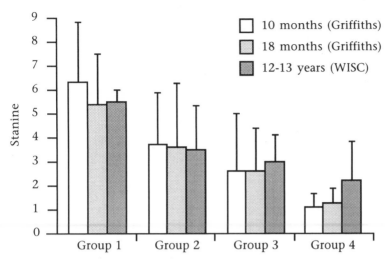

Figure 3. Comparison among mean Griffith's Mental Development scores (+ 1 s.d.) at 10 and 18 months and mean WISC-R IQ scores (+ 1 s.d.) at 12 to 13 years for children in different prenatal exposure groups.

information (see Figure 2). The remaining 2 children in this group also had pronounced difficulties in arithmetic. The children in the moderate group (group 2), scored low on the digit span subtest. The results of the Raven test confirmed those obtained using the WISC. Figure 3 compares data from the Griffith's Mental Development Test, obtained when the children were 10 and 18 months old, with the WISC-R IQ scores obtained when the children were 12 to 13 years old.

The Bender test results indicated that 10 children had a severe delay (more than three years) in the development of visual perception. Three of the five children with neonatally diagnosed FAS were in this group, as were five of the remaining nine children from group 3 and 4. Two children from group 2 had this type of severe delay according to the Bender test.

Two children (one from group 4 and one from group 2) met full criteria for Asperger syndrome according to Gillberg and Gillberg (1989).

Psychosocial situations for children and biological mothers. Three of the 25 biological mothers had died before the follow-up data were collected.

Sixteen of the 24 children lived in foster homes at the time of follow-up. Eleven of these 16 children had been taken into care

TABLE 1. Children's living situations according to mothers' drinking during pregnancy.

Group: n =	1 (4)	2 (7)	3 (8)	4 (5)	Total (24)
Biological parent	3	4	0	1	8
Foster home	1	3	8	4	16

TABLE 2.Children's schooling according to mothers' drinking during pregnancy.

Group: n =	1 (4)	2 (7)	3 (8)	4 (5)	Total (24)
Regular school	4	3	0	0	7
Special education	0	4	5	2	11
ESN *	0	0	3	3	6

*Education for the Intellectually Subnormal.

before 18 months of age. Eight children were still living with their biological parents (Table 1).

Most of the fostered children had been living in environments unsuitable for small children before the time of fostering, with biological mothers who abused alcohol, changed partners often, and were unable to provide a sense of security for the children because of their own personal problems.

The biological mothers of 16 children had received therapeutic assistance in their own homes. At the time of the interview, nine mothers were still abusing alcohol, and at least five mothers were consuming drugs. Group 1 mothers, those who stopped their alcohol consumption early in pregnancy, had best succeeded in changing their social situation. Most of them still were taking care of their children. Other forms of support included day nurseries, housing, summer accommodations, and long-term sick leave benefits. Fifteen mothers had been in psychiatric treatment clinics for alcohol abuse.

Interviews with the principal caretaker suggested that the children's most significant problems were a lack of impulse control and bursts of aggression. The children seemed not to realize the consequences of their own behavior and demanded much more attention than normal children. Several foster parents felt that they needed more support in their role as parents to these children. Support had been granted from different authorities such as social services, pediatric clinics, child and adolescent psychiatric clinics, preschools, and day nurseries.

Children's school difficulties. Of the 24 children for whom information about the school situation was available, six attended schools or classrooms for mentally handicapped children. Eleven received some kind of special education support from the school, and seven attended normal classrooms. In the first two groups, 11 children received special education in mathematics and the Swedish language, and nine had a personal assistant (Table 2).

Interviews with the teachers made it clear that a majority of the children had problems learning mathematics and Swedish. They had poor attention and showed little perseverance. These children understood instructions more easily in a smaller group. Some of them readily made new friends, but had a hard time keeping them.

The Retrospective Study of Outcomes in Relation to Environmental Upbringing

We conducted another study to look at the importance of the postnatal environment of the children in relation to outcomes. Data for this retrospective study were collected from medical charts; social security files; interviews with social workers, psychologists, medical doctors, teachers, nurses; and direct observations from school health centers.

Three groups of children were formed according to estimated mental capacity based on test performance and school performance:

Group 1: Children with estimated normal intelligence (n = 50);

Group 2: Children with estimated borderline mental retardation (n = 33);

Group 3: Children with estimated mild to severe mental retardation (n = 12).

Central nervous system (CNS) dysfunction and neuropsychological problems in the children were indicated by hyperactivity, impulsiveness, distractibility, temper tantrums, short memory spans, concentration difficulties, perservations, perceptual disorders, and specific learning disabilities. Three of these symptoms were required for a child to be classified as having neuropsychological problems or CNS dysfunction.

Psychosocial problems in the children were defined as difficulties in relating to others, aggressiveness, poor self-confidence, psychosomatic symptoms, insecurity, anxiety, truancy, juvenile delinquency and drug abuse. Three of these symptoms were required for a child to be classified as having psychosocial problems.

The children were assigned to four groups according to the social environment in which they were raised:

Group A: Children raised in a single foster home or adoptive home after only one intervention;

Group B: Children raised in a foster home after several interventions and changes of home;

Group C: Children raised mainly in the biological home after several temporary interventions;

Group D: Children raised in the biological home with no interventions.

Children in groups A and B were not raised mainly by their biological parents in contrast to the children in groups C and D who were raised mainly in their biological homes.

Classification of mental capacity, neuropsychological problems and psychosocial problems were made independently of the assignment to social environment group. Twenty-two of the 30 mothers in this study had themselves been raised in an environment where extensive use of alcohol was part of their life and/or came from broken, poor, or unhappy homes. The children of 16 of these 22 women were taken into custody.

Results

Table 3 shows the relationship between type of rearing environment and child outcome for the 95 children in the retrospective study. The mean age of the children at the time of investigation did not differ between groups, nor was any difference in sex distribution found. The mean ages and gender distributions of groups were comparable.

Children raised in foster homes or adoptive care (groups A and B) had fewer psychosocial problems than had children living in their biological homes (groups C and D), with significant differences found between groups A and C, groups A and D, and groups B and C. No significant differences between groups were found in mental capacity or neuropsychological problems. However, among the children with neuropsychological problems, no child placed in foster care before six months of age had acquired psychosocial problems.

There were no significant differences in psychosocial problems across the three mental capacity groups or between groups with and without neuropsychological problems.

TABLE 3. Outcome of children in relation to different types of childhood environments.

Group: n =	A (29) n (%)	B (29) n (%)	C (24) n (%)	D (13) n (%)	Total (95) n (%)
Mental capacity					
Normal	16 (55%)	14 (48%)	12 (50%)	8 (62%)	50 (53%)
Borderline	10 (35)	9 (31)	11 (46)	3 (38)	33 (35)
Mild/severe	3 (10)	6 (21)	1 (04)	2 (15)	12 (13)
Neuropsychologic problems	14 (48)	16 (55)	12 (50)	5 (38)	47 (49)
Psychosocial problems	7 (24)	13 (45)*	20 (83)**	9 (69)*	49 (52)
Mean age at follow-up	14.2	14.7	14.9	13.5	14.3

* p <.05 compared with A. **p<.01 compared with A.

Discussion and Conclusions

The results presented here focus on the multiplicity of problems to which children of alcoholic mothers are exposed. The influence of both prenatal and postnatal factors reveals a wide spectrum of impact on both the physical and psychological development of these children.

The follow-up study shows that a majority of the children exposed to abuse levels of alcohol in utero had attention deficits, motor control problems, or both, in pre-adolescence. Specific learning disorders also were very common, and mild mental retardation occurred in about one of six cases. Other researchers (Lemoine & Lemoine, 1992; Steinhausen, 1995; Streissguth, Aase et al., 1991; Streissguth, Clarren, & Jones, 1985) have reported similar results from follow-up studies in the USA, France, and Germany.

In accordance with the results of our previously published studies, the children displayed higher rates of disturbance and more severe disturbance when their mothers had abused alcohol throughout the pregnancy. The children whose mothers ended their alcohol consumption before the twelfth week of gestation all developed normally and did not show conspicuous difficulties in school.

The retrospective study shows that developmental retardation, perceptual difficulties, attention deficits, and pre- and postnatal growth retardation were not significantly reduced in children placed in good foster homes early in life. This strongly suggests that these disturbances are of prenatal origin. Good foster homes evidently cannot fully compensate for the prenatally acquired handicap.

Even though early fostering did not appear to eliminate the harmful effects of exposure to alcohol in utero, foster care seems to be the most favorable alternative for children whose biological mothers, despite vigorous attempts at psychological support, continue to abuse alcohol and have severe personal psychological problems. Children prenatally exposed to alcohol who remain in biological families with continued alcohol problems appear to be doubly handicapped. In addition to their prenatal and primary damage, the continued risk of experiencing psychosocial problems is present. Our clinical impression suggests that placement in a foster home leads to improved performance and a better quality of life for affected children, but normalization does not occur. We have the impression that the fostered children were better able to cope with their difficulties than were those who remained in their biological homes.

Primary and Secondary Disabilities in Fetal Alcohol Syndrome

Ann Streissguth, Helen Barr, Julia Kogan and Fred Bookstein

Introduction

In 1973, Kenneth Lyons Jones and David W. Smith, dysmorphologists at the University of Washington Medical School, identified a "similar pattern of craniofacial, limb, and cardiovascular defects associated with prenatal onset growth deficiency and developmental delay" in eight unrelated children, of three ethnic groups, born to chronic alcoholic mothers (Jones, Smith, Ulleland, & Streissguth, 1973, p. 1267). The distinctive pattern of malformations indicated that the damage was prenatal. In a second report, three more infants were identified, and the first necropsy on such a patient "disclosed serious dysmorphogenesis of the brain," (p. 999) which the authors thought might be responsible for some of the functional abnormalities and joint malpositions seen in the syndrome. The naming of this syndrome as Fetal Alcohol Syndrome (FAS) put the emphasis squarely on the presumed etiology and brought international attention to this phenomenon (Jones & Smith, 1973). Among the letters that came to David Smith was one from Paul Lemoine of Nantes, France, who in 1968 had published, in a regional French medical journal, a study of children born to alcoholic mothers who had similar features and behaviors.

From the start, both groups of investigators were fascinated with the unusual behaviors of these children who looked alike (although they were not related) and who behaved alike in a hyperactive and unfocused manner. In 1974, Jones and colleagues, using data from the National Perinatal Collaborative Project (NPCP) reported that 44% of the children of chronic alcoholic mothers identified during pregnancy had borderline to moderate mental retardation (defined as an IQ of 79 or below) when examined at 7 years of age. Of the same

This paper was supported by the Centers for Disease Control and Prevention Grant # R04/CCR008515.

children, 32% had enough abnormal features from the physical examination alone to suggest the Fetal Alcohol Syndrome. In a carefully matched comparison group selected from over 50,000 other women and children in the NPCP study, fewer than 10% of the other children had IQ scores below 79, and none had the physical features of FAS.

In 1978, Clarren and colleagues presented additional evidence of alcohol-related Central Nervous System (CNS) damage. Neuropatholgic findings on four human neonates exposed to large amounts of ethanol at frequent intervals during gestation revealed that "all four brains displayed similar malformations stemming from errors in migration of neuronal and glial elements," (p. 64). Two had hydrocephalus and only two of the four were diagnosed as having the Fetal Alcohol Syndrome from external criteria. They concluded: ". . . the brain alterations may be the only distinct abnormality produced by in utero ethanol exposure," (p. 64). Since 1978, children who had some but not all the features of FAS have been referred to as having Fetal Alcohol Effects (FAE) (Hanson, Streissguth, & Smith, 1978) or Possible Fetal Alcohol Effects (PFAE) (Clarren & Smith, 1978). Recently there have been suggestions that the terminology should be reconsidered (Aase, Jones, & Clarren, 1995; Stratton, Howe & Battaglia, 1996).

Within four years of the naming of Fetal Alcohol Syndrome, experimental studies of laboratory animals were published demonstrating that alcohol is teratogenic and can produce malformations from prenatal exposure (Chernoff, 1977; Randall, 1977). By 1978, 245 patients with Fetal Alcohol Syndrome had been reported in the medical literature, and FAS was described as the "most frequent known teratogenic cause of mental deficiency in the western world" (Clarren & Smith, 1978). It also was recognized by this time that prenatal alcohol exposure produces a whole spectrum of effects. FAS is the most clearly definable, but not necessarily the most prevalent.

By the mid-1980s, it was apparent that the physical features of FAS were less characteristic after the onset of adolescence. Patients with this disorder whom we had watched grow up in Seattle had far more life problems than would be expected solely on the basis of their mental retardation or delayed development. Furthermore, as more patients were evaluated, it was clear that there were many children with the full features of FAS who did not legally qualify as "mentally retarded", and so, had trouble obtaining appropriate services (Streissguth, Clarren, & Jones, 1985). Many of the children without the physical manifestations of FAS who were born to alcohol-abusing mothers likewise had cognitive and adaptive behavior problems similar to those of children with FAS (Streissguth, Randels, & Smith, 1991).

Public policies to prevent FAS and other prenatal effects of alcohol began almost as soon as alcohol was clearly identified as a teratogen. In 1981, the Surgeon General of the U.S. recommended that women not drink alcoholic beverages during pregnancy or when planning a pregnancy. Congress passed legislation in 1989 to mandate warning labels on all alcohol beverage containers sold in the U.S. that included a warning against drinking alcohol during pregnancy.

FAS and FAE have been recognized for the past 20 years as major known causes of developmental disability. Yet, it is only in the past 10 years that the lifelong implications of these disabilities have been recognized. Follow-up studies in four countries have demonstrated the continuing adverse effects of prenatal alcohol exposure into adolescence and adulthood (Aronson & Olegård, 1987; Lemoine & Lemoine, 1992; Majewski, 1993; Spohr, Willms, & Steinhausen, 1994; 1993; Steinhausen, Willms, & Spohr, 1994; 1993; Streissguth, Aase et al., 1991; Streissguth, Clarren, & Jones, 1985). In 1992, in recognition of this problem, the Centers for Disease Control and Prevention (CDC) through the National Center for Environmental Health, Disabilities Prevention Program, issued a request for proposals. The research study described in this chapter was undertaken in response to that request. The aim of this study has been to build a prevention information base fundamental to the amelioration of secondary disabilities in patients with FAS and FAE.

For the purposes of this study, *primary* disabilities are defined as functional deficits that reflect the CNS dysfunctions inherent in the FAS or FAE diagnosis. *Secondary* disabilities are those that arise after birth and presumably could be ameliorated through better understanding and appropriate interventions.

The study had three main goals:

1. To document the occurrence and range of secondary disabilities that are associated with FAS and FAE. These include mental health problems, disrupted school experiences, trouble with the law, confinement, inappropriate sexual behavior, and drug/alcohol problems.

2. To determine the risk and protective factors associated with these secondary disabilities. A *risk factor* is a characteristic or condition that increases the odds of a particular disability occurring. A *protective factor* is a characteristic or condition that decreases the odds of a secondary disability occurring. *Universal* risk or protective factors are those that apply to all six of the secondary disabilities in which we are most interested. *Specific* risk or protective factors are those that

apply to only some of the six, or that increase the odds of some secondary disabilities while decreasing the odds of others. *Intrinsic* risk or protective factors are those that present in the child at the time of birth; *extrinsic* factors are those that could conceivably be modified by the social or institutional environment in which the child is situated after birth.

3. To develop a brief Fetal Alcohol Behavior Scale (FABS) so that state/community agencies may identify patients with probable FAS/FAE. This goal is addressed elsewhere (Streissguth, Barr, & Press, 1996).

Methods

Diagnostic Criteria

Fetal Alcohol Syndrome (FAS) is diagnosed by the co-occurrence of three primary characteristics: growth deficiency, a characteristic pattern of abnormalities primarily observable in the face, and some manifestation of Central Nervous System (CNS) dysfunction. The definition of CNS criteria used here is in keeping with that originally used by Clarren and Smith (1978) and is *not* wholly consistent with the modification suggested by the recent IOM (Stratton, Howe, & Battaglia, 1996) report for diagnosing FAS. Over the years, a small number of children had been diagnosed PFAS (possible or probable FAS). This term was applied to borderline cases in which, for instance, CNS criteria and facial features were characteristic, but the growth deficiency was marginal, or in which the CNS criteria and growth deficiency were characteristic and the face was "almost" characteristic. For this report, PFAS and FAS are combined. Fetal Alcohol Effects (FAE) and PFAE (possible or probable FAE) are terms that have been used clinically to apply to individuals who manifest some, but not all of the characteristics of FAS, but were exposed prenatally to significant alcohol. The terms FAE and PFAE, as they have been used by Seattle dysmorphologists since 1974, *are* consistent with the new diagnostic category of ARND (Alcohol Related Neurodevelopmental Disabilities) suggested by the IOM (Stratton, Howe, & Battaglia, 1996). For this report, the FAE and PFAE categories are combined.

In the present study, a diagnosis of FAS is assigned to patients who have (1) a clear history of prenatal alcohol exposure; (2) certain dysmorphic features such as short palpebral fissures, a pattern of flat midface, smooth and/or long philtrum, and thin upper lip; (3) growth retardation for height and/or weight below the 10th percentile of normal growth; and (4) central nervous system (CNS) dysfunction, as manifested by microcephaly, developmental delay, hyperactivity, attention and/or memory deficits, learning difficulties, intellectual deficits, motor problems, neurologic signs, and/or seizures. A diagnosis of FAE or PFAE is attributed to those who have a clear history of prenatal alcohol exposure and CNS dysfunction, but who do not manifest all of the physical features of FAS. All diagnostic evaluations were performed by physicians trained in dysmorphology and genetics.

Ascertainment

The 661 patients in this study represent a gradually accrued group that began with the first patients diagnosed FAS in 1973 by Jones and Smith and ended with those who came to the University of Washington FAS Diagnostic Clinic between 1993 and 1995. The patients were largely ascertained through clinical referral across a 22 year period. Diagnosis was by a small, homogeneous group of dysmorphologists, all trained by David W. Smith at the University of Washington Dysmorphology Unit. The sample includes, but is not limited to, all those available from the following published studies: 11 patients from the two 1973 Lancet papers describing FAS (Jones & Smith, 1973; Jones, Smith, Ulleland, & Streissguth, 1973); 20 and 17 patients respectively, from the first two FAS follow-up studies (Streissguth, Herman, & Smith, 1978); 8 patients from the 10 year follow-up study of the first 11 patients diagnosed with FAS (Streissguth, Clarren, & Jones, 1985); Northwest sample only (n = 31) of the first FAS follow-up study of adolescents and adults (Streissguth, Aase, et al., 1991a); 40 patients from the test-retest IQ study of adolescents and adults (Streissguth, Randels, & Smith, 1991); and 24 patients from the FAS genotype study (Faustman, Streissguth, Stevenson, Omenn, & Yoshida, 1992). Patients from southwest Indian reservations who were included in earlier reports (LaDue, Streissguth, & Randels, 1992; Streissguth, Aase et al., 1991; Streissguth, LaDue, & Randels, 1988) are not included in the current report because their recruitment and follow-up were not comparable to those patients in the Northwest. Out of the full 661, 61% were diagnosed in 1993 or later at the University of Washington FAS Diagnostic Clinic, directed by Sterling Clarren, who was responsible for two-thirds of their diagnoses. These patients were primarily from the Pacific Northwest.

The University of Washington FAS Diagnostic Clinic was established with primary funding from CDC in January 1993. Patients are referred to the FAS clinic by concerned caregivers such as physicians, parents, teachers, or caseworkers. Referral typically is a response to cognitive or behavioral problems; these must also be a confirmed or suspected history of prenatal alcohol exposure. As many more patients apply than can be seen, priority is given to those whose biologic mothers are living and known to be in the area, and to those whose profile of behavioral problems suggests FAS. See Clarren and Astley's chapter.

Recruitment

All clients from the FAS Diagnostic Clinic who were diagnosed FAS, PFAS, FAE, or PFAE were invited to participate in this secondary disability study. The study, which was approved by the University of Washington Human Subjects Review Committee, was explained to the families by our patient advocate. A Confidentiality Certificate was obtained from the Public Health Service to further protect the patients and their families. Consent from both patient and caregivers was obtained, for participation in the study, for use of photographs, and for release of information from schools, hospitals, etc. Patients from our other FAS research projects who met the diagnostic criteria were also notified about the new study and asked to participate wherever they could be located. Over a four year period, all these caregivers were contacted for information on past and current patient status, secondary disabilities, and risk and protective factors. Reports of psychological evaluations conducted for research purposes were provided upon request to the patients or their caregivers. In case of a crisis call, patients were referred to appropriate community agencies and professional local services.

Samples

Of the 661 patients in this study, 473 were sampled for analysis of primary disabilities and 415 were sampled for analysis of secondary disabilities. The two samples overlap; some patients are in both samples. All patients were diagnosed either FAS, FAE, PFAS, or PFAE as described above. Although the two samples are not entirely nested, the referral source, the diagnosing physician, and date of diagnosis are comparable for the two samples. The primary disabilities sample includes patients three years old and older; the secondary disabilities sample includes patients six years old and older.

60% of the secondary disabilities sample were white, 25% Native American, 7% black, 6% Hispanic, and 2% Asian and other. 57% were male. 37% were diagnosed FAS, the rest; FAE or PFAE. 39% of the subjects were between 6 and 11 years; 39% 12 to 20 years; and

22% 21 to 51 years old. Informants for the 415 Life History Interviews (see below) were surprisingly varied. 33% were adoptive mothers, 17% biological mothers, and 12% foster mothers. The rest were other relatives, legal guardians and others.

Primary Disabilities Sample (IQ): Tests Administered

Patients were administered an age-appropriate Wechsler IQ Test: the Wechsler Preschool and Primary Scale of Intelligence-Revised (WPPSI-R), the Wechsler Intelligence Scale for Children-Revised (WISC-R), or the Wechsler Adult Intelligence Scale-Revised (WAIS-R) (Wechsler, 1981; 1974; 1967). The Wide Range Achievement Test-Revised (WRAT-R) (Jastak & Wilkinson, 1984) was also administered individually to each patient. The Vineland Adaptive Behavior Scale (VABS) (Sparrow, Bella, & Cicchetti, 1984) was administered to a caretaker or person who knew the patient well, usually at the time the IQ and achievement tests were administered. Testing was carried out primarily at the Fetal Alcohol and Drug Unit (FADU) or in patients' homes or schools.

From the WPPSI, WISC-R, and WAIS-R, the present analyses used the full scale IQ score, the Verbal Scale IQ score (VIQ), the Performance Scale IQ score (PIQ), and the 11 Subtest Scores. WISC-III full scale IQ scores, corrected for comparability with the WISC-R, were used for 11 patients who either could not be seen at our lab for testing or who had been tested at their schools on the WISC-III within the prior year, so were not eligible for retesting. From the WRAT-R, we used the Standard Scores (SS) for Reading, Spelling, and Arithmetic. From the VABS we used the Standard Scores from the Adaptive Behavior Composite (ABC) and the Standard Scores for Socialization, Communication, and Daily Living Skills.

Secondary Disabilities Sample: Life History Interview (LHI)

The Life History Interview (LHI) was developed for this study to evaluate patients of any age and any degree of disability. The focus of the LHI, administered by telephone to caretakers/informants of the patients during the third year of the study, was on the kinds of secondary disabilities and risk and protective factors that characterize these patients.

The LHI is a structured evaluation of ten major areas of possible long-term functional covariates or consequences characteristic of patients diagnosed with FAS/FAE: (1) household and family environment; (2) independent living and financial management; (3) education; (4) employment; (5) physical abuse, sexual abuse and domestic violence; (6) physical, social and sexual development; (7) behavior management and mental health issues; (8) alcohol and drug use; (9) legal status and criminal justice involvement; and (10) companionship and parenting. These areas of concern were explored in terms of past and current patient status, secondary disabilities, and possible risk and protective factors.

450 separate questions are organized to provide the interviewer with clear visual guides for accurate coding. Most questions require the interviewer to code a choice from an available list of responses. Other questions permit open-ended responses, which were transcribed verbatim and coded later. Validity ratings by the interviewer follow each section of the LHI. A section is coded "questionable" if the informant did not know the patient well, seemed guarded, seemed confused and/or contradicted himself/herself, seemed to be biased, seemed hostile, did not understand or speak English very well, or seemed mentally handicapped.

Seven interviewers were trained in administration and coding procedures by the project director, who was regularly available to address queries. Each completed interview was reviewed by the team of interviewers, and coding consensus was reached for any items under contention. Finally, all coded interviews were reviewed by the project director before they were submitted for data entry.

The LHI took, on average, 70 minutes to administer (range, 18 to 215 minutes.) Interviews took longer to administer when they involved older patients or those with a greater number of secondary disabilities. Interview length was not related to sex, race, or alcohol-related diagnosis of the patient.

Most caregivers felt that the LHI covered major areas of the patient's functioning, in terms of prevalent problems, possible environmental buffers, and assessment of service needs. Many caregivers stated they felt that the data generated from this interview, once disseminated to the service agencies and community advocates, would help them provide better care for their children with FAS/FAE.

Quantifying Data Across the Life Span

The data summarized here pertain to the whole life course of the patient. For example, a patient who was 16 years old at the time of the LHI might have been diagnosed with FAS when three years old and given an IQ test when five years old. In addition, some questions on the LHI assess the age of onset for many outcomes and break out other problems, such as school problems, by developmental age.

The Final Report (Streissguth, Barr, Kogan, & Bookstein, 1996) is replete with graphics describing the findings and the subcategories involved in each secondary disability.

A set of 21 possible risk and protective factors was examined through an analysis of odds ratio plots across the first six secondary disabilities. When risk and protective factors involved continuous scores (as in 1, 4, 5, and 8 below) the cut point for risk versus protective factors was defined as the sample median.

The "odds ratio" of a risk or protective factor for a single secondary disability is the ratio of two ratios. One is the odds of the disability for those *having* the factor, the other the odds of the disability for those *not having* the factor. In symbols, if SF is the count of those having both the disability and the factor, SG the count of those having the disability but not the factor, TF the count of those having the factor but not the disability, and TG the count of those having neither the factor nor the disability, then the odds ratio is (SF × TG) / (SG × TF). For the Final Report to the CDC (Streissguth, Barr, Kogan, & Bookstein, 1996), data were framed in the positive perspective of odds of avoiding secondary disabilities; those odds ratios are the inverse: (SG x TF) / (SF x TF). For risk factors, this is smaller than 1.0; for protective factors, it is larger.

Summary of Findings

Findings on Primary Disabilities

The primary disabilities associated with FAS/FAE were examined in 473 patients who ranged in age from 3 to 51 years. Those with FAS (n = 178) had an average IQ of 79, average reading, spelling, and arithmetic standard scores of 78, 75, and 70, and an average Adaptive Behavior standard score of 61. Those with FAE (n = 295) had an average IQ of 90, average reading, spelling, and arithmetic standard scores of 84, 81, and 76, respectively, and an average Adaptive Behavior score of 67. (For both IQ and Adaptive Behavior, a score of 100 is normal.)

Findings on Secondary Disabilities

Secondary disabilities and risk and protective factors were assessed primarily from the LHI. The LHI was administered to all available caretakers/informants of 415 patients with FAS/FAE. The patients ranged in age from 6 to 51 years with a median of 14.2 years.

Six main secondary disabilities were studied.

- *Mental Health Problems (MHP)*, defined as ever having gone to a psychotherapist or counselor for a mental health problem or having any one of a long list of mental health problems, was by far the most prevalent secondary disability, experienced by over 90% of the full sample (6 and over).

- *Disrupted School Experience (DSE)*, defined as having been suspended or expelled from school or having dropped out of school, was experienced by 60% of patients (12 and over).
- *Trouble With the Law (TWL)*, defined as ever having been in trouble with authorities, charged, or convicted of a crime, was experienced by 60% of the patients (12 and over).
- *Confinement (CNF)*, including inpatient treatment for mental health problems or alcohol/drug problems, or ever having been incarcerated for a crime, was experienced by about 50% of the patients (12 and over).
- *Inappropriate Sexual Behavior (ISB)*, including having been reported to have repeated problems with one or more of 10 inappropriate sexual behaviors or ever having been sentenced to a sexual offenders' treatment program, was noted for about 50% of the patients (12 and over).
- *Alcohol/Drug Problems (ADP)*, defined as having been in treatment for an alcohol or drug problem or as having alcohol and/or drug abuse problems, was noted for about 30% of the patients (12 and over).

In an effort to determine how many patients became self-sufficient as adults, two additional secondary disabilities were evaluated for the 90 patients who were at least 21 years old (median age 26 years):

- *Dependent Living (DPL)*, characterized about 80% of the sample (21 and over).
- *Problems With Employment (PWE)*, characterized about 80% of the sample (21 and over) (Streissguth, Barr, Kogan, & Bookstein, 1996).

Only seven of the 90 adults in this sample live independently *and* without employment problems.

Males have higher rates of Disrupted School Experience, Trouble With the Law, and Confinement than do females. Otherwise, rates of secondary disabilities are nearly equal across the sexes. Patients 12 years and older have a higher rate of all secondary disabilities except Mental Health Problems than younger patients. Compared to patients with FAS, those with FAE have a *higher* rate of all secondary disabilities, except Mental Health Problems.

Adults with FAE have as high a rate of Dependent Living as do those with FAS, but a somewhat *lower* rate of Problems With Employment, which may reflect their higher IQ level.

A diagnosis before 6 years of age (which characterized 11% of those 12 years old and older), is a strong protective factor for all secondary disabilities except Mental Health Problems.

Findings on Risk and Protective Factors

Eight universal protective factors emerged from the analyses of patients 12 years old and older. In order of their strength, they are:

1. Living in a stable and nurturant home for over 72% of life;
2. Being diagnosed before the age of 6 years;
3. Never having experienced violence against oneself;
4. Staying in each living situation for an average of more than 2.8 years;
5. Experiencing a good quality home (10 or more of 12 good qualities) from age 8 to 12 years;
6. Being found eligible for DDD (Division of Developmental Disabilities) services;
7. Having a diagnosis of FAS (rather than FAE);
8. Having basic needs met for at least 13% of life.

Odds of Mental Health Problems and Odds of Disrupted School Experience are reduced primarily by the universal protective factors.

The rate of Trouble with the Law is related to all the universal protective factors, most notably DDD eligibility for services.

Confinement also is related to the universal protective factors, especially living in a stable and nurturant environment, and being diagnosed prior to age 6.

Odds of Inappropriate Sexual Behavior are reduced by all universal protective factors.

Alcohol and Drug Problems have one specific protective factor in addition to universal protective factors: having lived with an alcohol abuser *less* than the median for the group, which was 30% of life.

Odds of Dependent Living are increased fourfold for patients who had an IQ score of 70 or below, or a VABS score below 65. Other strong intrinsic risk factors for Dependent Living are a high FABS score and being male. An extrinsic factor that is protective against Dependent Living is having a diagnosis before 6 years of age. (Home quality and stability, basic needs met, living with alcohol or drug abusers, or having FAS versus FAE were not associated with Dependent Living as an adult.)

Odds of Problems with Employment are increased more than two to fourfold by having an IQ score of 70 or below, having a VABS score below 65, and being diagnosed FAS rather than FAE. Some universal factors are also protective against Problems with Employment, namely, an early diagnosis, longer time in a stable and nurturant home, longer duration in each household, and not being a victim of violence.

A low IQ score (70 and below) is a protective factor for Disrupted School Experience, Trouble With the Law, Confinement, and Alcohol and Drug Problems. IQ level has little relationship to Mental Health Problems or Inappropriate Sexual Behavior, but low IQ is obviously a risk factor for Dependent Living and Problems With Employment.

Across the full age spectrum of 415 individuals with FAS/FAE, Mental Health Problems characterize 94%, followed by Inappropriate Sexual Behavior (45%), Disrupted School Experience (43%), and Trouble with the Law (42%). As anticipated, the most protective environmental factors *against* secondary disabilities are living in a stable and nurturant home of good quality, not having frequent changes of household, and not being a victim of violence. Two intrinsic characteristics are associated with a *higher* level of secondary disabilities: having FAE rather than FAS and having an IQ above 70 rather than below. Special attention should focus on patients with these "risky" characteristics in order to prevent secondary disabilities.

The 90 adults studied (21 years and over) had an 83% rate of living dependently and a 79% rate of problems with employment. The most important environmental factor protecting against these two secondary disabilities is an early diagnosis, suggesting that families and communities may have provided special help and opportunities for those patients identified early in life as FAS/FAE.

In fact, an early diagnosis is a strong universal protective factor for all secondary disabilities, yet only 11% of these individuals with FAS/FAE were diagnosed by age 6. Every effort should be made to provide an early diagnosis for every child with FAS and FAE. Applying for and receiving eligibility for services from the state s Division of Developmental Disabilities (DDD) is also a strong protective factor for most secondary disabilities. The services provided by DDD appear to be both useful and necessary for many patients with FAS/FAE who do not now qualify.

Violence against individuals with FAS/FAE occurred at an alarming rate: 72% had experienced physical or sexual abuse or domestic violence. Being a victim of violence was a strong risk factor for Inappropriate Sexual Behavior, increasing the odds fourfold. Children and adults disabled by FAS/FAE must have better protection against violence and their families may need special training and guidance about intervention with Inappropriate Sexual Behavior.

Thirty females with FAS/FAE had given birth to a child. Of these, 57% no longer had the child in their care; 40% were drinking during pregnancy; 17% had children diagnosed FAS or FAE; and an additional 13% had children who were suspected by the informants of having FAS/FAE. Special advocacy services for these high-risk mothers who themselves have FAS/FAE and special attention to their birth control needs and child care needs should be a top priority (see chapter by Grant, Ernst, Streissguth, & Porter).

In addition,

- The correlations reported may or may not be causative. They nonetheless suggest courses of action that may be beneficial both to these patients, and ultimately to society.

- Many environmental influences that appear beneficial for patients with FAS/FAE are, of course, good for all people—all the more reason that society should safeguard them for people born with a birth defect, particularly a "hidden" birth defect like FAS/FAE.

- Seven of the eight universal protective factors are extrinsic and presumably could be modified by society.

- Efforts to intervene with alcohol-affected children should proceed simultaneously with efforts to prevent future children from being born with FAS and FAE.

Recommendations Deriving from the Findings

1. Develop statewide networks of local FAS/FAE Diagnostic Clinics coordinated with local community service providers, to facilitate proper labeling of the child's organic brain damage as early as possible (see chapter by Clarren and Astley).

2. Develop a coordinated system of parent and citizen education centers, and a system for ongoing in-service training programs for all relevant service providers. These should focus on strategies for improving the patient's quality of life, facilitating appropriate, long-term placement in a good quality home, and providing the appropriate life skills and job skills training.

3. Develop a state inter-agency network to facilitate detection, diagnosis, and provision of services to this population. The network should include representatives from key state and private agencies and parent groups. There should be an "FAS/FAE Coordinator" within each agency. State agencies of health, mental health, schools and special education, the juvenile and criminal justice, and alcohol and drug abuse treatment should be involved in this effort.

4. Fund research on methods to quantify the central nervous system impairments associated with FAS/FAE in order to develop clinically-useful diagnostic tools for the neurobehavioral effects of prenatal alcohol exposure. This should facilitate diagnosis of alcohol-affected individuals without facial dysmorphology or growth deficiency, and should permit response to their service needs before the onset of secondary disabilities.

5. Develop and test modification of eligibility criteria for the Division of Developmental Disabilities. Enhancing eligibility for case management, job coaching, and supervised housing should reduce the level of costly secondary disabilities among individuals with FAS/FAE who are unable to live and work independently, but are now unable to get appropriate services whenever they have an IQ above 70 or lack the full FAS diagnosis.

6. Fund a model long-term residential/job training program for youth and adults with FAS/FAE.

7. Mandate the full disclosure of medical and mental health histories when placing a child in foster or adoptive placements, and provide education and training on FAS/FAE and appropriate support services to all people raising such children, including biological parents.

8. Prevent the birth of additional children with FAS/FAE by providing appropriate treatment, advocacy and long-term birth control options to women with alcohol problems.

Also, of course, we need to work to reduce the prevalence of the primary disabilities that are the ultimate cause of the secondary disabilities reviewed here: (1) Expand alcohol/drug inpatient treatment programs for women and their children, and (2) Fund state-wide networks of Birth to 3 Advocacy programs for working with the highest-risk mothers abusing alcohol/drugs during pregnancy (see chapter by Grant, Ernst, Streissguth, & Porter), and (3) make long-term family planning options freely available for women with alcohol problems.

People with FAS and FAE have an unacceptable level of secondary disabilities that severely impairs their quality of life and is extremely costly to society. The low level of societal protection and support given to people with FAS and FAE and their families is unacceptable and further compromises their lives. They should be given an appropriate level of societal protection and support. To do this, their primary disabilities must be better understood by families, service providers, and by society at large. (See Kleinfeld and Wescott, 1993, for accounts of parents and teachers responding to the needs of individual children with FAS and FAE. See Streissguth, 1997, for first-hand accounts by people with FAS and FAE and their caretakers, and strategies for families and communities for developing systems for better detection and advocacy across the lifespan.)

The permanent, organic brain damage of people with FAS and FAE is often "hidden" in that it often does not conform to current system guidelines for providing services, such as having a low IQ score, a debilitating physical handicap, serious mental illness, or even an FAS face (and diagnosis). By understanding the devastating secondary disabilities that characterize most individuals with FAS/FAE, and by understanding the intrinsic and extrinsic risk and protective factors that exacerbate or ameliorate these disabilities, we should be able to improve the quality of life for people with FAS and FAE and their families, and reduce costs to society.

Development of the FAS Diagnostic and Prevention Network in Washington State

Sterling Clarren and Susan Astley

Introduction

It has not yet been demonstrated that stories and warnings in the media about the adverse impact of drinking alcohol during pregnancy lead directly to a reduction in the incidence of Fetal Alcohol Syndrome (FAS) and related disorders. However, it has become clear to us that every time a widely viewed piece on FAS appears in the press or on television, there is a sharp increase in requests for appointments for FAS diagnosis. Parents seem to recognize their own children's difficulties in the descriptions of patients with FAS and wonder if FAS is, at last, the elusive answer to the enigma that is their child.

We began to receive requests for FAS diagnoses in the late 1970s after the first major articles on FAS had been published (Clarren & Smith, 1978; Hanson, Jones, & Smith, 1976; Jones, Smith, Ulleland, & Streissguth, 1973) and the first major campaign to improve maternal awareness and decrease alcohol use in pregnancy had been mounted (Little, Streissguth, & Guzinski, 1980). For many years, we attempted to serve these patients' diagnostic needs through referrals to existing clinics at Children's Hospital and Medical Center, in Seattle, Washington. Some patients were evaluated in diagnostic clinics such as Medical Genetics, Dysmorphology, Neurology, or Developmental Disabilities. Others were followed in chronic care clinics like the Craniofacial or Neurodevelopmental Programs.

The feedback we received from both patients and faculty was generally neutral to negative. None of these medical settings seemed to meet the needs of many of the patients. The families recognized almost immediately that whether or not they received a specific diag-

This paper was supported in part by the Centers for Disease Control Cooperative Agreement # U84/CCU008707-04 and the March of Dimes Birth Defects Foundation.

nosis , they had sought much more. They really wanted help with management across four large domains: medical, psychiatric/psychologic, educational, and social, with recommendations for specific interventions by specific individuals in their locality. Funding was almost always a major concern. Most of our faculty were capable of making an accurate medical diagnosis of FAS, but no program was prepared to evaluate and appropriately treat or refer the patients in a comprehensive fashion for the myriad of functional problems that led to the evaluation in the first place.

By the late 1980s it became clear that a new clinic was needed to address the long term management needs of patients debilitated by alcohol teratogenesis. The clinic had to be prepared to evaluate patients of all ages and to handle different types of problems in clients of different ages — because FAS produced ongoing needs across the life span. In infants and children below the age of three years or so, the diagnosis was more important for future planning than for any specific intervention at that time. In children of preschool and primary school years, academic and behavioral problems were a major issue. Academic problems were seen as more important, although in middle school years concern over behavioral problems generally outweighed concern over the ongoing academic issues. In older teens and adults, problems of employment, relationships, and independent living were often the primary concerns. Frequently, the patients' specific problems did not meet specific criteria for help as defined by the schools or the social welfare system.

However, if the birth mother of an affected child was able to have more children and was still drinking, she was at high risk to have other children with alcohol-related problems and was at high risk to have alcohol-related health problems of her own. Issues of alcohol abuse and addiction existed in families of patients of all ages, expressed through the mother's feelings about herself, the other family member's feelings about her, and concern for the patient's own susceptibility to alcohol abuse and addiction. The identification of young FAS patients needed to be attached to a program that would reach out and help the birth mothers. This issue had to be identified and dealt with specifically because it affected all other interventions.

It seemed reasonable that the new clinic would work well if it was based on a traditional multi-disciplinary developmental model that would be responsive to patients and caregivers with varying needs in a context of available local services. We found that such a new clinic for FAS patients was not easy to establish. The majority of the assessments and treatments that were needed were not medical, but social, educational, psychologic, or related to addictions. As long as the clinic was run from a hospital base and billed as a medical service, the financial reimbursement was so low that the clinic was not viable. Beyond fee for service, no other means of funding a service clinic was readily available to us. Unfortunately, if a clinic is never established because there is no funding mechanism, then the value of the clinic cannot be demonstrated and the financial "Catch-22" cannot be understood and corrected.

In 1990, we responded to a Request for Proposal from the Centers for Disease Control and Prevention (CDC). The CDC was looking for innovative approaches to the primary prevention of FAS. We suggested that an immediate reduction in the incidence of FAS could be accomplished by identifying women who had had an FAS child. If these women could be helped to become clean and sober through any subsequent pregnancies, then pregnancies at the highest risk for producing infants with FAS could be avoided. But who were these women, and what factors in their lives needed to be understood for an effective intervention to work? To this time, there have been no published reports describing the lives of mothers of FAS patients as a group in the general population of the United States. It was clear from our personal experience and the general literature that FAS patients frequently did not live with their birth mothers. A clinic that would make regular, accurate, and consistent diagnoses of FAS and related conditions would demonstrate that the mothers could be found. The birth mothers could then be interviewed as a first step in developing a focused intervention plan.

This project was funded by the CDC. We are now in the fourth year of a five year study. The project allowed us to create the FAS Diagnostic Clinic at the University of Washington's Center for Human Development and Disability, which was the beginning of the development of the FAS Diagnostic and Prevention Network of Washington State.

The CDC funding permitted us to schedule the clinic to meet one day per week. We found that four or five patients could be assessed in a clinic day, and between 160 to 180 patients could be evaluated in a year. Our waiting list grew steadily. At times, 500 or more names were on the waiting list. Clearly, we could never see all of the applicants. The fact that so many families requested appointments, and were willing to wait months to be seen, underlined our previous impression that while numerous facilities were available to assess FAS in the context of some specific discipline or another, and that while most of these families had availed themselves of some of these services, the families still did not believe that their children had been appropriately understood or directed to appropriate services.

We worked with the March of Dimes Foundation for Healthier Babies to establish two FAS Network sites (in King and Snohomish Counties). These sites were based on our clinic model at the University of Washington, the concept of multiple funding sources, and perceived community interest by professionals and families. Our group provided training and data management and the local staff were responsible for patient assessment and treatment planning. At that same time, the Washington State Legislature, responding to lobbying from concerned parents, wished to develop a model for helping with the perceived unmet needs of patients with FAS and their families. We suggested to a state senator, who was drafting legislation, that our FAS Network idea might make sense for the state. The concept was adopted in Senate Bill 5688 that became state law in 1995. The law provided for the development of several additional sites, which currently is ongoing. Funding was made available for development, training, and data management. The sites remain responsible for finding the resources needed to cover patient care costs.

All clinics will function similarly to the clinic established at the University of Washington. The structure of that clinic is described below.

The Clinic

Staff

The *primary staff* are the core group of professionals needed for diagnosis and treatment plan development for all patients. The ideal team comprises individuals from six disciplines: medicine, psychology, speech and language pathology, social work, public health nursing, and family advocacy. The first three members are largely responsible for the assessments necessary to make the diagnosis and develop the treatment plan; the latter three members more often are responsible for helping to implement the plan.

The *secondary staff* are a larger group of professionals that can be called on to consult in specific cases, but would not necessarily be needed in all cases. Staff members might include (but would not be limited to) medical subspecialties like psychiatry, neurology or genetics, alcohol treatment counselors, educators, educational psychologists, behavioral therapists, family therapists, lawyers, and parent support groups.

Referral Process

Referrals are accepted from any primary sources including physicians, teachers, psychologists, social service agencies, the courts, and the families themselves. In order to gauge the appropriateness of the referral, the family is asked to complete an extensive questionnaire. This document asks for information in all areas that will be pertinent to the diagnosis, including gestational history and gestational exposures to drugs and alcohol, basic genetic historical information, and descriptions of medical, social, educational, and behavioral problems. Photos are requested.

The returned questionnaires are reviewed at weekly meetings and the patients are placed in one of three groups:

Group A. The patient has a documented history of exposure to alcohol in utero and there are physical anomalies and behavior problems present. A diagnosis of FAS, a related condition, or another birth defect syndrome is likely.

Group B. The patient has a documented history of alcohol exposure in utero or physical anomalies and/or behavioral problems so that a diagnosis of FAS or a related condition still may be reasonably considered.

Group C. The patient has no documented history of alcohol exposure in utero and no physical anomalies. Although the patient's behavioral problems might be just as serious as are those of patients in groups A and B, it is unlikely that the clinic will be able to link the etiology to ethanol teratogenesis or reach out to a birth mother in hope of preventing subsequent cases.

Patients in groups A and B are scheduled to be seen at the clinic. Because the clinic currently is funded as a research tool aimed at finding the mothers of FAS patients, patients in group A with the highest likelihood of having FAS, and a birth mother still known to be living in Washington State, are given the highest priority. Conversely, patients in group C are sent a letter suggesting that they be evaluated in another setting. Specific alternate settings are suggested when appropriate.

Clinic Process

The patient's evaluation can be divided into five distinct "phases:"

Phase 0: Collection of old records. Phase 0 occurs between the time the referral is accepted for an appointment and the actual clinic day. Most patients who are evaluated in our program already have had multiple evaluations including medical, psychological, educational, and social-welfare reviews. During this waiting period, the clinic coordinator and possibly the family advocate work with the family to identify and locate copies of these materials.

Phase 1: Clinical assessments. This phase involves the collection of new data by team members. At a minimum, this will include an interview with the family and the patient, and a physical exam emphasizing dysmorphological and neurological conditions. If the old records do not contain current and appropriate psychometric test results, then such tests will need to be obtained as well. The most helpful tests usually are IQ measures, tests of academic performance, tests of language usage, and tests of adaptive ability.

Phase 2: Case conference. The staff meets as a whole to discuss the diagnosis(es) and the etiologies of the diagnosis(es), and to develop an initial treatment plan. The family then is invited into the session, the situation is clarified, and the final treatment plan is developed with input from the family.

Phase 3: Debriefing. The family then meets with a single member of the staff, usually the psychologist, to discuss the emotional impact of the clinical day and the diagnosis. We have found that this phase is critical in helping the family to use the information from the clinic in a positive way. After having been "talked at," families need time to "talk back" and process the situation.

Phase 4: Staff closure. After the debriefing period, the psychologist usually needs to finalize the case with the rest of the staff and arrange for any follow-up with team members that was suggested in Phase 3. This also is an appropriate time to insure that all records have been completed.

Diagnostic Schema

The definition of FAS has changed little in the last twenty years (Clarren & Smith, 1978; Rosett, 1980; Sokol & Clarren, 1989). The condition is typified by growth deficiency, a characteristic set of facial features, and evidence of prenatal alteration in brain function such as microcephaly from birth, neurologic problems without postnatal antecedents, or complex patterns of functional disability that cannot be explained or understood solely in terms of postnatal experiences. The condition is distinctive and can be readily separated from normal and almost all other birth defect syndromes by trained observers (Astley & Clarren, 1995; Clarren et al., 1987). The history of alcohol exposure in gestation is not part of the clinical criteria for the diagnosis of FAS, but rather the history of alcohol supports the diagnosis.

For the trained clinician, there is little difficulty in making the diagnosis of FAS when the abnormalities in growth, face, and brain are all extreme, and the alcohol exposure history is conclusive and substantial. But the features of the condition are not dichotomous; the clinical features and, indeed, the history of alcohol exposure itself each range along a separate continuum from normal to clearly abnormal. Accurately and fairly characterizing intermediate conditions has posed difficulties. To date, clinicians have not agreed on a simple diagnostic schema to deal with the gradations in exposure and in effects.

In our clinic, several diagnostic terms initially were used to deal with this problem. These are:

FAS with confirmed history of alcohol exposure. These patients met the full published diagnostic criteria of growth deficiency; a full and characteristic set of minor facial anomalies including short palpebral fissures (more than two standard deviations from the mean), and a complex lower facial malformation sequence typified by flat philtrum, thin upper lip and apparent flattening of the midface just medial to the alae of the nose; and evidence of organic brain damage including structural, neurological, or functional stigmata. In these cases, there is clear evidence of exposure to alcohol during gestation by reliable report. Other malformations also may be found and are noted, but do not affect the final diagnosis.

FAS without a confirmed history of alcohol exposure. These patients have the same phenotypic findings as above, but no history of alcohol can be confirmed because the family of origin is not available, the birth records are sealed, or there is some similar situation. (We have never seen a patient with the full FAS phenotype and a confirmed negative history for alcohol exposure in gestation, but if such a patient would be found, they would not have FAS, but rather would be referred to as having an "FAS phenocopy.")

Atypical FAS. These patients have a phenotype that very nearly is complete for FAS and have a confirmed history of alcohol exposure. We place patients in this category when they have the full facial stigmata and brain changes of FAS, but lack growth deficiencies, or when they have growth deficiencies and brain changes of FAS, and most, but not all, of the facial anomalies. Specifically, they have short palpebral fissures and two out of three of the lower facial features, or all of the lower facial features and palpebral fissures that are more than one but less than two standard deviations from the mean. (In the past, we referred to this patient group as "possible FAS" or "partial FAS". Both of those terms proved problematic for patients, as we found that service providers interpreted "possible" FAS to mean an uncertain diagnosis and "partial" FAS to mean a milder form of the disorder.)

"Possible fetal alcohol effects" or *"alcohol-related neurodevelopmental disorder."* These terms both refer to a needed category(ies) for classifying patients exposed to alcohol in utero, but the terms themselves are less than ideal. The category broadly includes patients with some of the physical, cognitive, and/or behavioral problems that are among the problems seen in patients with FAS and an alcohol exposure history that would support high risk for alcohol teratogenesis. "Fetal alcohol effect" (FAE) was a term that was developed for research studies in humans or in animals when a teratogenic result (that was not full FAS) was clearly associated with alcohol exposure (Clarren & Smith, 1978). This term was needed because alcohol does have broad teratogenic impacts, especially on the brain, that are not necessarily related to obvious physical anomalies. The term "possible FAE" was proposed for clinical work as an entry on the differential diagnosis because the findings in these patients were generally nonspecific for alcohol teratogenesis and alcohol exposure could not be seen with certainty as the only cause. Although the term has been widely used by the public, it has been troubling or confusing to professionals who felt the term was used as a final diagnosis, rather than as a possible diagnosis, and that it overstated the established relationship between cause and effect (Aase, Jones, & Clarren, 1995). Further, what "effect" was being described? The term "alcohol-related birth defects" was proposed as an alternative (Sokol & Clarren, 1989). This term was not widely used because it did not seem to be appropriate to describe patients with functional brain dysfunction of probable organic origin as having a birth defect. Even more recently, the term "alcohol related neurodevelopmental disorder" has been suggested for this category name (Stratton, Howe, & Battaglia, 1996). The term is better in emphasizing the neurodevelopmental nature of the "effect," but this new term, in the end, continues to be problematic in its inherent link of etiology and outcome in the same phrase when the relationship between alcohol exposure and the likelihood of organic brain damage are each on a continuum from minimal to extreme, and the relationship between the two ranges from clinically very likely to clinically very unlikely. Better terminology is still needed and we are actively working on this problem at this time.

Financial Support

Much of the evaluation for FAS and related conditions, and most of the recommendations, are not medical, but rather social, educational, or involve mental health, so it is not wholly surprising that the costs are frequently not borne by medical insurers in total. We are finding that there are two ways to address this problem: build the model within an existing system while avoiding duplication and develop multiple funding sources. Our clinic sites are establishing themselves within existing facilities in their communities such as public health departments, alcohol treatment facilities, and neuro-developmental programs within a children's hospital. These organi-zations have pre-existing infrastructures that provide space, support systems, billing mechanisms, and natural linkages to other needed services. The development of various funding streams includes cash and in-kind contributions from private or government grants, fee-for-service contractual relationships for screening and diagnosing clients within a specific system (such as adoption agencies, schools, courts, and corrections), and support from managed care providers who do not wish to fully gear up to provide these diagnostic services themselves. In-kind support includes coverage of salaries for any of the clinic staff who serve the client population as part of their exist-ing job (especially educational psychology, social work, and public health nursing). In-kind support also can include both professional and nonprofessional volunteers.

Results

In the first three years of clinic operation (January 8, 1993 to December 31, 1995), 1,839 requests were received for appointments to the FAS Diagnostic Clinic at the Center for Human Development and Disability. Of these, 816 families completed and returned the "New Patient Information Form," and 511 patients were evaluated. Among the 511 patients evaluated, 103 (20%) met the criteria for FAS (with or without confirmed exposure) or atypical FAS, and another 304 (60%) were placed in the FAE group. Males were more likely to have an FAS or FAE diagnosis. Sixty-six (64%) of FAS patients were male, and 168 (55%) of FAE patients were male (Table 1).

The racial background of the patients (Table 2) generally reflected the racial mix of Washington State, with the exceptions that patients with Native American ancestry were somewhat over-represented, and patients with Asian ancestry were under-represented.

Children with FAS and FAE generally did not live with their birth mothers (Table 2) . Only 15% of FAS patients and 21% of FAE patients lived with their birth mothers. The birth fathers or other family members cared for each group about 20% of the time. Fifty-five percent of the patients were in foster or adoptive care and 10% were living independently or in group homes. Few were incarcerated.

TABLE 1. Patient ages and gender by diagnosis.

Patient Diagnosis:	FAS (n = 103)	PFAE (n = 304)	Other (n = 104)	All (n = 511)
Age (yrs) at visit				
mean (s.d.)	10.4 (7.5)	10.2 (7.1)	9.9 (8.6)	10.2 (7.5)
{min—max}	{0.3—46.3}	{0.6—50.9}	{0.2—48.2}	{0.2—50.9}
Gender				
M:F (% male)	66:37 (64)	168:136 (55)	54:50 (52)	266:223 (56)

TABLE 2. Selected patient characteristics by diagnosis.

Patient Diagnosis:	FAS (n = 103)		PFAE (n = 304)		Other (n = 104)		All (n = 511)	
	n	(%)	n	(%)	n	(%)	n	(%)
Race								
Caucasian	58	(56)	145	(48)	54	(52)	257	(50)
Black	9	(9)	29	(10)	10	(10)	48	(9)
Am/Alask Indian	21	(20)	79	(25)	19	(18)	119	(23)
Other	14	(14)	51	(17)	21	(20)	86	(17)
Unknown	1	(1)	0	(0)	0	(0)	1	(1)
Primary caretaker								
Birth mother	16	(15)	62	(21)	22	(21)	100	(20)
Birth father	8	(8)	27	(9)	6	(6)	41	(8)
Other family member	14	(13)	35	(12)	16	(15)	65	(13)
Foster care	28	(27)	99	(32)	28	(28)	155	(30)
Adoptive care	26	(26)	59	(20)	25	(24)	110	(22)
Other	10	(10)	22	(7)	7	(6)	38	(7)
Accompanied child to clinic								
Birth mother	17	(17)	72	(24)	28	(27)	117	(23)
Birth father	9	(9)	23	(8)	6	(6)	38	(7)
Other family member	9	(9)	37	(12)	12	(12)	58	(11)
Foster parent	31	(30)	86	(28)	24	(23)	141	(28)
Adoptive parent	26	(25)	59	(19)	24	(23)	109	(22)
Other	11	(10)	27	(9)	9	(9)	48	(9)

Approximately 90% of the patients paid for the assessment through Medicaid funding.

Although all of the patients had been assessed by at least one physician and many had seen numerous physicians and other professionals, the diagnosis of FAS had only been suggested in 4 of the 103 patients who met diagnostic criteria. Another 10 patients had been previously diagnosed as FAS but did not meet our diagnostic criteria.

Relatively few patients with FAS had medical problems that required follow-up. Nearly all needed coordinated services involving psychiatry (drug therapy for ADHD and/or mood), educational/vocational planning, behavioral therapy, family counseling and guidance, and drug and alcohol abuse counseling for older patients.

Discussion

Why is there a need for clinics uniquely devoted to patients with Fetal Alcohol Syndrome and related conditions? In part, the answer seems pragmatic. Our experience would suggest that the patients and their families do not seem to believe that their needs are met elsewhere. In part, the answer lies in the fact that the term "Fetal Alcohol Syndrome" actually identifies two patients. The "fetal alcohol" part of the term is relevant to etiology and is important in recognizing that the birth mother is a patient who is highly vulnerable to produce more affected children and to be judged as a poor caretaker of her current children. The diagnosis should direct us to her so that we can support her in her attempts at sobriety for her sake, and for the sake of her children and her unborn children. The "syndrome" part of the FAS term is relevant to the child who is likely to have complex cognitive and behavioral problems requiring the help of an appropriate team made up largely of educational and mental health professionals. Accurate diagnosis and treatment planning not only is needed for primary prevention and secondary disability prevention, but also is needed for epidemiological studies. Without accurate diagnosis and prevalence figures, the success of prevention programs cannot be gauged nor can appropriate budgets for intervention be calculated.

Our clinic model offers a comprehensive approach to the needs of both mothers and children. The clinic sites will be located conveniently throughout the state. Diagnosis will be consistent and defensible. Treatment planning will be comprehensive. In time, we can determine what services are available, or not available, available but not affordable, and effective or not effective. Clinics will aggressively, but sympathetically, reach out to birth mothers and help to identify factors that need to be addressed so that reductions in recurrent cases of FAS and FAE will occur. Finally, the clinics will be an important tool for surveillance programs.

If FAS screening is to be done, individuals who screen positive need to be evaluated for an accurate diagnosis and an appropriate treatment plan. Social groups and agencies in our state, including juvenile rehabilitation, foster care, and several Native American communities, already have approached the Network and asked to become clients of the system. Photographic screening of facial shape

(Stratton, Howe, & Battaglia, 1996) should be used to select the appropriate patients for clinical assessment. The development of the FAS Diagnostic and Prevention Network is just underway. At this time, two of the FAS Diagnostic and Prevention Network sites are open and meeting once every other month, and four additional sites are in the training phase. The groups are all enthusiastic and committed. We are very optimistic that the program will be well-received within communities and will offer a much needed service.

Although the Washington State Legislature has only funded us to develop sites within Washington, the system could easily be expanded to a regional or national schema. This should be considered within a year or so, based on the success of the state-wide model.

End note: To obtain a copy of Astley and Clarren's manual, *Diagnostic Guide for Fetal Alcohol Syndrome and Related Conditions: The 4-Digit Diagnostic Code,* University of Washington, March 1997, contact: Fetal Alcohol Syndrome Diagnostic and Prevention Network, Children's Hospital and Medical Center, 4800 Sand Point Way N.E., CH-47, Seattle, WA 98105, or phone (206) 526-2206.

Assessment and Treatment of an Adult with FAS: Neuropsychological and Behavioral Considerations

Kathleen Dyer, Gregory Alberts and George Niemann

Introduction

Fetal Alcohol Syndrome (FAS) is the leading known cause of mental retardation in the United States (Abel & Sokol, 1987). The incidence of FAS is nearly twice that of Down's syndrome, and nearly five times that of spina bifida. FAS refers to a recognizable pattern of abnormalities observed in children exposed to large quantities of alcohol before birth. It is characterized by the presence of 1) intrauterine growth deficiency; 2) a pattern of specific anomalies, including characteristic facial features; and 3) central nervous system dysfunction, evidenced by developmental delay, hyperactivity, problems in attention and learning, and intellectual deficits (Clarren & Smith, 1978).

Individuals with FAS also display a common cluster of behavioral characteristics, including high levels of sociability, impulsiveness, hyperactivity, poor attention span, lack of inhibition, out of context conversation, and poor social judgment (Steinhausen, Nestler, & Spohr, 1982; Streissguth, 1992; Streissguth, LaDue, & Randels, 1988). These behaviors repeatedly lead these individuals into dangerous situations and, as such, caretakers and teachers express the constant need for monitoring these individuals at all times. While it is imperative to develop an understanding of why these behavior problems occur so that positive behavioral support can be provided for these individuals, there is a relative absence of data in the scientific literature to address these problems.

One method to accomplish an improved understanding of FAS related behaviors is to conduct a functional analysis, which is an assessment process for gathering information regarding possible environmental factors that contribute to the occurrence of the problem behavior (O'Neill, Horner, Albin, Storey, & Sprague, 1990). In addition to an analysis of environmental variables, it would also be important to determine if neuropsychological variables contribute to the problem behavior. That is, given that individuals with FAS demonstrate central nervous system dysfunction (Stratton, Howe, & Battaglia, 1996), it would be important to determine the manifestations of this dysfunction as it contributes to the problem behaviors seen in these individuals.

We therefore conducted the following in-depth study of one individual with Fetal Alcohol Syndrome as a first step in understanding these behaviors. The following experimental questions were asked:

1. Do environmental variables affect problem behaviors characteristic of individuals with FAS?

2. How do deficits in neuropsychological functioning contribute to problem behaviors characteristic of individuals with FAS?

This chapter will describe the assessment data that were gathered on this individual to answer these questions, and describe necessary treatment components that were designed to support this individual that are consistent with the assessment results.

Neurobehavioral Assessment

Michael (a pseudonym), an 18-year-old individual with Fetal Alcohol Syndrome, was the participant in this study. Michael lived with eight other adolescents in a campus-based group home setting at Bancroft Inc., in New Jersey. Bancroft is an organization that provides a full continuum of comprehensive residential, educational, and vocational support for individuals with developmental disabilities and brain injury (see chapter by Hess and Nieman). Michael also received educational and vocational supports in the community.

He was described by caregivers and physicians as having secondary consequences of FAS, including learning disabilities, attention-deficit hyperactivity disorder, and conduct problems. He was described as having "poor impulse control" and an "inability to comprehend the consequences of his behavior." He was receiving Imipramine daily for treatment of his attentional disorder.

To develop an understanding of the possible variables contributing to Michael's behavior, two assessments were administered: The Functional Analysis of Problem Behavior: A Practical Assessment Guide (O'Neill, Horner, Albin, Storey, & Sprague, 1990) and the Halstead-Reitan Neuropsychological Test Battery for Adults (HRB; Reitan & Wolfson, 1992).

Functional Analysis of Behavior

The Functional Analysis of Problem Behavior involved three strategies for collecting information about possible environmental variables controlling Michael's behavior: (1) conducting a functional analysis interview; (2) directly observing Michael in his every day environments; and (3) manipulating his environment in order to directly observe the effects on behavior. These procedures are described in detail elsewhere (O'Neill, Horner, Albin, Storey, & Sprague, 1990), and will be summarized here.

The functional analysis interview was conducted with three caregivers who had worked extensively with Michael in his educational, residential, and vocational settings. The following behaviors were reported to be of concern: hyperactivity (motor restlessness and excessive activity), stealing, leaving the area, music disruption, off-task behaviors, talking out of context, harassing peers, and exaggerated or delusional speech.

The staff reported that Michael's behaviors seemed to occur particularly when staff attention was reduced, when there were too many distractions in his environments, and when structured programming was not in place. They also reported that he exhibited these problems when he became confused, and when he was with new staff and with certain peers who also have problems with distractibility.

In order to observe problem behaviors in a number of different contexts, direct observations of problem behaviors were conducted in three different settings. Two of the settings were those where Michael spent the majority of his time: his classroom and his vocational site—a restaurant where he worked as a dishwasher. The third setting was a small room with a minimal amount of distractions, where he was undergoing neuropsychological testing.

During the direct observation sessions, Michael was observed continuously during 10-second intervals. During each interval, a recording was made of the occurrence or nonoccurrence of problem behavior, and important setting events that were present during the behavior. The problem behaviors included out of seat/area, out of context talking, bragging, off-task behavior, and fidgeting. The setting events included novel independent activity (e.g., classroom worksheets), routine independent activity (washing dishes), caregiver directed activity, caregiver attention, peer attention, and transitions. At the end of each observation session, the percentage of 10-second intervals during which Michael exhibited problem behavior was calculated.

The pattern of behavior that emerged from analysis of the direct observations was that Michael engaged in lower rates of problem behavior in situations that had a high degree of structure. Therefore, the following Structure Gradient was developed, where points were given for three components characteristic of high structure. These components were:

a) Acquired routine - a repetitious task that Michael had learned to proficiency.

b) Adult-imposed structure - a task in which the adult specifies the exact response required at least once every five minutes.

c) Low distraction - an environment free of distracting activities such as people talking or engaged in activities.

The amount of structure in each activity is presented in Table 1. This table shows that Michael was involved in settings that had various degrees of structure.

Figure 1 shows the percent of time Michael displayed behaviors during direct observation in different settings. The percent of time Michael displayed problem behavior is presented on the ordinate, and the Structure Gradient is presented on the abscissa. The results show that Michael exhibited high amounts of problem behavior in low structured environments.

The results of the functional analysis interview and direct observation suggested that Michael demonstrated increases in problem behavior in less structured environments. This hypothesis was more rigorously tested by conducting systematic environmental manipulations of the effects of structure on Michael's problem behaviors.

In order to accomplish the environmental manipulations, a *high structure* and *low structure* condition were manipulated in Michael's natural environment (his gym class) in the context of a reversal design (Dunlap, Kern-Dunlap, Clarke, & Robbins, 1991). In the *high structured* condition, Michael was instructed to follow a specific routine in the gym. Specifically, the instructor would first model the behavior desired with a verbal description (e.g., "Throw the volleyball so it hits above the line on the wall"). The instructor would then tell Michael to do exactly what he did. In the nonstructured condition, the instructor would give Michael a more general instruction (e.g., "I want you to practice volleyball skills today"). As in the direct observations above, Michael was observed continuously, and the occurrence of problem behavior was recorded during 10-second intervals. At the end of each observation session, the percentage of 10-second intervals during which Michael exhibited problem behavior was calculated.

TABLE 1. Structure gradient for activities that Michael was engaged in during direct observations. A point (+) was assigned for each component characteristic of high structure, and a (0) was assigned when the component characteristic of high structure was not present.

Antecedent	Acquired Routine	Adult Structure	Low Distraction	Structure Gradient
Low-structured classroom	0	0	0	0
High-structured classroom	0	+	0	1
Work	+	0	0	1
Testing	0	+	+	2

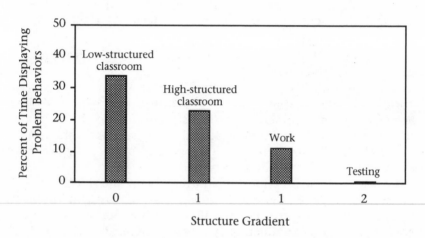

Figure 1. Percent of time Michael displayed problem behaviors during direct observation in different settings.

The results of the environmental manipulations are presented in Figure 2. As can be seen from the figure, Michael's problem behaviors were consistently higher in conditions involving less structure. These data more strongly support the hypothesis that lower amounts of problem behavior occur in situations with a high degree of structure for Michael.

Halstead-Reitan Neuropsychological Test Battery for Adults

Our neuropsychological examination of Michael consisted of an administration of the Halstead-Reitan Neuropsychological Test Battery (HRB; Reitan & Wolfson, 1992), a comprehensive and thoroughly validated set of standardized tests for assessing human brain-behavior relationships (Hartlage, 1987; Parsons, 1986). The

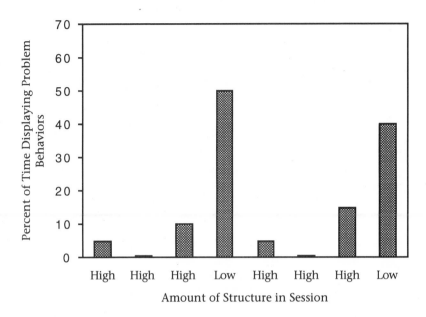

Figure 2. Percent of time Michael displayed problem behaviors during eight high- and low-structured activity sessions.

HRB consists of a number of different procedures that allow for a comprehensive sampling of various brain-related skills ranging from abilities which are very basic (e.g., tactile perception) to those that are more advanced (e.g., conceptual problem solving). The HRB procedures evaluate "input" (i.e., stimulus reception via the sensory avenues), "central processing" (i.e., recalling, manipulating, and integrating information and generating inferences based on that information) and "output" abilities (i.e., execution of a motor or verbal response).

The core procedures of the HRB which were administered to Michael included the following:

Lateral Dominance Examination: A measure of handedness.

Finger Tapping Test: A measure of bilateral finger dexterity and speed.

Grip Strength: A measure of bilateral upper extremity grip strength.

Tactual Performance Test: A measure of complex psychomotor problem solving ability, interhemispheric transfer of learning, incidental memory, and memory for spatial information.

Sensory Perceptual Examination: A series of procedures which assess the integrity of simple to more complex stimulus input across tactile, auditory, and visual pathways.

Category Test: A measure of non-verbal logical reasoning and analysis, abstraction, concept formation, and memory.

Trail Making Tests, Parts A & B: Measures of sustained attention, divided attention, cognitive flexibility, and spatial analysis.

Seashore Rhythm Test: A measure of attention, registration, and immediate memory for complex auditory tonal patterns.

Speech Sounds Perception Test: A measure of attention, registration, and immediate memory for nonsense syllables.

Aphasia Screening Test: A series of tasks requiring naming, drawing (copying), spelling, reading, writing, arithmetic, word repetition, giving verbal explanations, naming body parts, and locating body position. Evaluates for signs which signal various dysphasias in language and visual/spatial systems.

Incorporated into the neuropsychological assessment battery are standardized measures of intelligence (Wechsler Adult Intelligence Scale [WAIS]) and academic achievement (Wide Range Achievement Test). Michael obtained a Full Scale IQ of 78 (Verbal IQ = 77; Performance IQ = 82) which placed him in the "borderline" range of intellectual functioning. He achieved academic achievement levels in reading (word pronunciation) at a 10th grade level. However, his ability to spell to dictation and to perform written calculations were measured at the 4th and 5th grade levels, respectively.

On the HRB, he obtained a Halstead Impairment index of 0.4. This value, which reflects the consistency (versus the severity) of impairment, indicated that his performance on three of the seven assessment measures with the highest sensitivity to brain damage fell beyond the cutoff score that distinguishes impaired from normal performance. In particular, he had a marked degree of deficit on three tasks that are most strongly associated with the integrity of diffuse, higher order neural systems distributed throughout the cortex. These variables included the Category Test, a measure of abstraction and reasoning, the Trail Making Test-Part B, a measure of divided attention, symbol recognition, and mental flexibility, and a memory component of the Tactual Performance Test, an "incidental" learning assessment reflecting Michael's recall of the test stimuli.

On the Aphasia Screening Test, Michael's performance revealed multiple pathognomonic signs (i.e., errors attributable almost exclusively to brain impairment) consistent with left and right hemisphere dysfunction. The left hemisphere signs included right-left confusion, central dysarthria (deficits in enunciating words), and dyslexia or visual word dysgnosia. The right hemisphere signs involved constructional dyspraxia (a deficit in the ability to deal with spatial relationships of a two- or three-dimensional nature).

Regarding neuropsychological strengths, Michael tested as having a number of areas of relative competence. He had low-average Performance IQ abilities. General "hands on" manipulation and problem-solving were within normal limits. His attention and concentration abilities (presumably with medication support and examiner-imposed structure) tested as within normal limits. He demonstrated very adequate sensory-perceptual abilities across visual, tactile, and auditory avenues. Comparative performances with each hand on simple motor output tasks (i.e., finger tapping and grip strength) revealed largely normal right-left (dominant/non-dominant hand) relationships on the measures.

In general, the test performances produced by Michael reflected an ability repertoire that showed considerable unevenness. His performances ranged from average or within normal limits on some tasks to degrees of deficit on other tasks that fell within moderate to severe levels of impairment. He generated normal level performances on the simplest and more fundamental or basic skill areas—namely motor output, sensory perception, attention/concentration, and manual problem solving using his hands. Many of these tasks were low in complexity, easy to execute, and the response was well specified and/or determined for him (e.g., finger tapping). As the task demands required more active thinking, careful observation, studying and discerning the important and essential features of a problem situation, thinking flexibly, and ultimately generating effective, plausible responses (e.g., abstract reasoning), he showed more moderate levels of deficit. Purely from a neuropsychological standpoint, this was an individual who "looked good" on a superficial level — in terms of general language, motor and sensory integrity, level of alertness and so on. However, when he had to impose some degree of organization on his environment — through studying, analyzing, remembering, and the like, that is, imposing structure and meaning to a situation — we found he had a significant degree of disability.

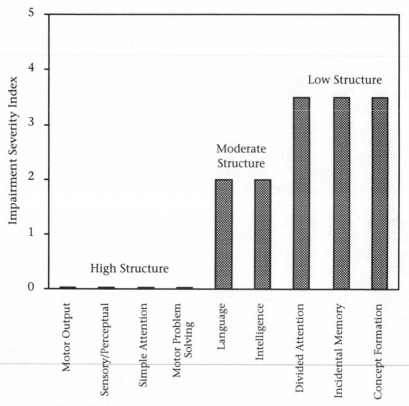

Figure 3. Michael's degree of impairment on neuropsychological assessments grouped by amount of structure of task.

Further, his pattern of test performances suggested that as the task demands became greater, i.e., when the requirements for both comprehending and responding to the test stimuli were increased and the structuring and organizing cues were less available (thereby requiring that he "impose" order and logic to the problem situation), there was an incremental deterioration in his performance.

This relationship between examiner-imposed structure and performance is reflected in Figure 3. General task areas of assessment as discussed above (e.g., motor output, language) are shown on the abscissa, and an impairment severity index is shown on the ordinate. On the severity index, 0 indicates no impairment, and 4 indicates severe impairment. The figure shows that in tasks involving a high degree of examiner-imposed structure, such as motor output and sensory/perceptual tasks, no impairment was seen. As the examiner-imposed structure decreased, the severity of impairment increased significantly.

In general, the particular ability structure of this individual is such that it predisposes him to experience a variety of problems in interpersonal and adaptive living domains. The area of greatest impairment for Michael and that which has broadest implications for his adaptive functioning concerns his critical reasoning abilities. When it comes to analyzing a situation, identifying critical elements that may prove useful in developing solutions, getting at the "heart" of the problem, and organizing several elements of information related to a particular problem, he has a substantial degree of deficit.

These brain-related impairments in reasoning are compounded by Michael's limited ability to self-monitor his behavior and, more importantly, to use feedback based on the effect his behavior has on his environment to generate alternate, more adaptive ways of responding. His very adequate performance on components of a psychomotor problem-solving task, when considered in light of his difficulties with abstraction and cause-effect reasoning, correspond with an impulsive, ill-considered, and an "act before one thinks" approach to dealing with day-to-day problems.

Further, Michael's (relatively) stronger verbal-based skills render him vulnerable to inflated expectations by others regarding his overall problem-solving and functional capacity. His verbal intelligence test scores (misleadingly) portray him as being more adept in executing real-time, practical, and creative problem-solving in the adaptive living sphere than in fact he is. Through this combined behavior analysis and neuropsychological assessment, we can conclude that this individual's neuropsychological deficits are not manifest in all situations, only those "complex" and minimally structured ones which require he impose order and meaning to the situation in order to behave adaptively.

Treatment

The results of this case analysis tie in with a growing body of literature on individuals with FAS. Specifically, these individuals are reported to have behavioral or cognitive problems that are thought to result from organic brain damage. These include attention problems (Nanson & Hiscock, 1990), learning disability — with better strength in reading than in math (Streissguth, Bookstein, Sampson, & Barr, 1993), and specific language deficits (Abkarian, 1992). Problems with reasoning and judgment are evidenced, as well as an inability to develop a logical approach to tasks (Stratton, Howe, & Battaglia, 1996).

The results of the above neurobehavioral assessment revealed that Michael's problem behavior varied as a function of environment, with increases in these behaviors seen in less structured environments. The neuropsychological assessment revealed a pattern of deficits that predispose Michael to behavior problems in low structured environments. This was found in Michael's residential environment, in which the behavior pattern continued with more serious behaviors, such as stealing and running away (behaviors that could not be directly observed in the above functional analysis). In Michael's residence at Bancroft, all the adolescents participated in a "level system," where the individual is provided with greater amounts of independence (and therefore less staff supervision and structure) contingent upon low rates of problem behavior. While this was a very effective system for the other adolescents with developmental disabilities with whom Michael lived, it proved to be problematic for him. Specifically, whenever Michael progressed to a level where he was given the opportunity to be unsupervised and independent, he would have an incident of serious problem behavior. These incidents involved elopement and therefore resulted in the involvement of law enforcement officials in the community.

This problem was also reported by Streissguth, LaDue, and Randels (1988), who reported the need for constant monitoring of activities and leisure time to keep individuals with FAS out of trouble. These authors also reported the difficulties individuals with FAS have in structuring their own behavior and the need to set external limits on their behavior.

The comprehensive program provided to Michael at Bancroft provided him with high amounts of adult structure and the opportunity to engage in acquired routines. He resided in an on-campus structured group home with a 1:2 ratio of staff to persons served. He was monitored 24 hours a day and was never in an unsupervised situation. In addition, he agreed to have staff support and instruction on how to manage his finances, due to his admission of having difficulty with impulsive spending. He worked at the local supermarket for 30 hours per week. In this setting, he engaged in acquired routines that involve bagging and moving cartons. He was in line of sight by the manager at all times.

The staff reported that with these supports in place, Michael was doing very well. However, due to the fact that he was 18 years old and due to be transferred to a funding source for adults, state funding agencies re-evaluated his need for state support. Because he was functioning in the "borderline" range of intelligence and he had no "hard neurological signs of impairment," the state mandated that he be discharged from Bancroft. This problem with receiving services has been evidenced in other states, due to the fact that FAS is not among the conditions identified as qualifying an individual for services (Bowman, 1994). After discharge, he moved into a boarding house in the community. Within a few weeks he was arrested for stealing a motor home and taking it for a "joy ride." Because the apparent theft occurred in the context of a prevailing probationary status, he went to jail, where he was at the time this case study was written.

Unfortunately, this outcome for Michael is not unlike those for many individuals with FAS. In a study of secondary disabilities for these individuals, Streissguth, Barr, Kogan and Bookstein (1996) found that over 60% of patients over twelve had been in trouble with the law (see the chapter by Streissguth and colleagues in this volume). These data point to the imperative to develop well-defined, structured services through private and public programs for individuals with FAS. They also indicate an urgency to continue additional systematic research studies to extend and replicate the findings of the current study and to validate the serious need for this type of support for these individuals.

A Study of Stimulant Medication
in Children with FAS

Jill Snyder, Jo Nanson, Richard Snyder, and Gerald Block

Introduction

In 1968 in France (Lemoine, Harouseau, Borteryu, & Menuet) and in 1973 in the United States (Jones, Smith, Ulleland, & Streissguth), researchers described a pattern of anomalies in children born to alcoholic mothers, which came to be labeled Fetal Alcohol Syndrome (FAS; Jones & Smith, 1973). Since then, it has been recognized that prenatal exposure to alcohol causes a spectrum of deleterious effects ranging from severe cognitive impairments, including mental retardation, to more subtle effects on behavior and learning ability, as well as the physical manifestations of the syndrome.

The diagnostic criteria for FAS were revised in 1989 (Sokol & Clarren) to include specific positive features in three diagnostic categories: growth, facial dysmorphology, and central nervous system (CNS) impairment. Although the physical manifestations of the syndrome are critical for diagnosis, it is the central nervous system defects that bring affected individuals to the attention of clinicians. If prenatal exposure to alcohol only caused individuals to be smaller and slightly dysmorphic, the syndrome would have little clinical significance. However, the prenatal insult to the developing central nervous system results in wide-spread behavioral and cognitive deficits that persist into adulthood (Habbick, Nanson, Snyder, Schulman, & Casey, 1996; Streissguth, Sampson, & Barr, 1989). The CNS deficits caused by prenatal exposure to alcohol can include varying degrees of mental retardation, learning disabilities, and attention deficit hyperactivity disorder (ADHD).

Of the behavioral deficits, ADHD is a frequent symptom in individuals with FAS at all developmental levels. ADHD frequently causes additional problems for the affected individual and his/her family.

The research presented here was completed as partial fulfillment of an Honors Degree in Psychology by the first author.

For example, Steinhausen, Willms, and Spohr (1993) reported that hyperkinetic disorders were the most frequent form of psychopathology in both preschool and school-aged children with FAS in Germany. More recently, Habbick and colleagues (1996) reported similar findings in an epidemiological study of FAS in a Canadian province over a 20-year span.

Problems with attention are not limited to children with FAS. Prenatal exposure to alcohol has been shown to moderate attention in children exposed to smaller amounts of alcohol in utero, who are not diagnosed as FAS. Streissguth, Barr, Sampson, and Bookstein (1994) followed a cohort of five hundred individuals for the first fourteen years of life. At four years of age, attention assessed by a vigilance task was adversely related to prenatal exposure to alcohol, when multiple confounding effects were controlled in the analysis. These deficits persisted in behavioral tasks of attention at 14 years of age.

ADHD is common in many clinical syndromes that cause a spectrum of developmental disability including autism and fragile-X (Hagerman, 1996) and is not unique to FAS. In order to assess the specific effects of ADHD on children with FAS, it is necessary to use carefully chosen control groups, not typically available for longitudinal studies, such as those described above. Nanson and her colleagues, in a series of cross-sectional studies, have compared the behavior of children with FAS to matched control groups and have found that problems with ADHD symptoms are common and persistent.

Nanson (1990) compared the behavior of twenty schoolchildren with FAS to the behavior of twenty age-matched children with pure ADHD and twenty normal children. The children with FAS had similar behavioral ratings to those of children with ADHD on a variety of parent measures including the Connors Abbreviated Rating Scale and the Child Behavior Checklist (CBCL), although the children with FAS were more cognitively impaired than were the children in the other two groups.

Nanson and Hiscock (1990) compared the performance of the same group of school-aged children with FAS to that of children with pure ADHD and controls using a variety of computerized tasks designed to measure attention and impulsivity, components of ADHD. They found that the children with FAS had similar deficits to those of children with ADHD and normal intelligence, but that children with FAS had additional motor learning deficits and an inability to make speed accuracy trades-offs when needed. They concluded that stimulant medications, which have been shown to be effective in treating children with ADHD, might also be effective in treating children with FAS.

Janzen, Nanson, and Block (1994) reported that a separate sample of fifteen preschoolers with FAS had significantly more behavior problems than had fifteen age-, IQ-, and race-matched controls, including problems with over-activity, impulsivity and short attention spans, the hallmarks of ADHD. This study was one of the few studies of children with FAS to employ race-matched controls, a critical factor as many children with FAS are of minority racial status.

ADHD is defined as a disorder of two behavioral domains; attention and hyperactivity-impulsivity (American Psychiatric Association, 1994). This model of ADHD follows earlier work by Douglas (1983) that identified three core components of the disorder; attention, impulsivity and hyperactivity. ADHD is typically diagnosed on the basis of parent or teacher rating scales such as the CBCL and the Connors scales. Less commonly, the components of the disorder are assessed directly using experimental tasks to define operationally the hyperactivity-impulsivity and inattention. The latter approach often is used in studies of treatment efficacy.

For example, Pelham and colleagues (1990) examined the effects of methylphenidate in children with ADHD who were participating in organized recreational activities. Seventeen boys diagnosed with ADHD ranging in age from seven to nine years participated in a double-blind, placebo-controlled study. The subjects underwent a series of four softball games during which several measures of attention were utilized. Hyperactivity and impulsivity were assessed in terms of the child's skills and ability to attend to critical factors in the game. Methylphenidate was shown to result in reduced hyperactivity and impulsivity during the softball games.

Similarly, Abikoff and Gittelman (1985) examined the effects of methylphenidate on the classroom behavior of children with ADHD. Twenty seven boys and one girl, ages six to twelve, underwent methylphenidate treatment for eight weeks and were compared with normal children. Methylphenidate was shown to be effective in reducing behavioral measures of impulsivity and hyperactivity in the classroom.

Although the treatment efficacy of stimulants for children with pure ADHD is well established, much less is known about the effects of stimulants for children with developmental disorders, even though the incidence of ADHD in these populations is high. Dickerson Mayes, Crites, Bixler, Humphrey, and Mattison (1994) argue that not enough research has been done investigating the effectiveness of these medications in multiply disabled children. In their study, 69 children with ADHD, ranging in age from 22 months to 13 years of age, underwent short-acting methylphenidate trials. Of these children, 36 had ADHD only and 33 had one or more additional developmental disorders (mental retardation, cerebral palsy, closed head injury or neurofibromatosis). The short form of the Conners rating scale was used. Methylphenidate was equally effective in reducing hyperactivity in children with or without additional developmental disorders, suggesting that the effects of methylphenidate are not limited to children of average intellectual ability.

Similar results were obtained by Aman, Marks, Turbott, Wilsher, and Merry (1991). A cross-over design was used to investigate the effects of methylphenidate and thioridazine (a major tranquilizer) in a group of school-aged children with ADHD and sub-average intelligence. A modified vigilance task was employed, similar to those used by Nanson and Hiscock (1990) and Streissguth and colleagues (1984). Methylphenidate but not thioridazine was shown to be effective in improving sustained attention in children with sub-average intelligence.

The proportion of ADHD children who improve with stimulant medications is not clear. Schatzberg and Cole (1991) estimated that 30% of children with ADHD prescribed dextroamphetamine sulfate, methylphenidate or pemoline show a high degree of clinical improvement and 40% show some modulation of behavior that may be of clinical importance. These authors also note that stimulants are thought to act by improving attention span and organizing behavior more effectively. Additionally, Simeon and Ferguson (1990) report that about 70% of children with ADHD treated with stimulants display overall improvement in attention, hyperactivity and impulsiveness. Data for children with developmental disabilities and ADHD is not available. Although Nanson and Hiscock (1990) suggested that stimulant medications might be helpful for children with FAS, and anecdotal evidence suggests that it is widely used with this population, there is no experimental evidence for its efficacy in FAS populations.

The purpose of this study was to investigate the effects of stimulant medication in children with FAS who also had been diagnosed as having ADHD. Specifically, we predicted that stimulant medication would result in improved attention in terms of faster reaction times and fewer errors of omission on the vigilance task; decreased impulsivity, in terms of higher scores on the underlining task; and less hyperactivity in terms of lower scores on the parent questionnaires compared to placebo conditions.

Method

Participants

The sample consisted of eleven children with FAS between the ages of six and 16 years (mean age, 9.7 years) from the Alvin Buckwold Child Development Program at the Kinsmen Children's Center in Saskatoon, Canada. These children were drawn from a database of individuals with FAS followed by this clinic. The development of this database has been described elsewhere (Habbick et al., 1996) and will not be described in detail here.

Twelve subjects participated initially, but one subject was at a very low developmental level and was not able to complete the tasks, in either the drug or placebo conditions and was eliminated from the study. Seven boys and four girls had been previously diagnosed with FAS in accordance with the criteria outlined in Sokol and Clarren (1989). In addition, all children had a positive maternal history for alcohol abuse. All subjects also fulfilled the diagnostic criteria for ADHD in accordance with the DSM-IV (American Psychiatric Association, 1994).

All participants were taking stimulant medications previously prescribed by the child's developmental pediatrician. Eight of the subjects had been prescribed methylphenidate, two pemoline and one dextroamphetamine sulfate. All children were judged by parents and teachers to have a positive response to stimulant medications prior to the onset of the study.

The parents of the participants initially were contacted by mail to explain the purpose and requirements of the study. If they expressed an interest in participating, they were contacted by phone to set up testing times. One family contacted declined to participate. All participants and parents of natural or adopted children were required to complete a consent form before they were included in the study. For children who were under the legal guardianship of the province, signed consent from the child's social worker was obtained. Families of participants living outside of the general area of Saskatoon received financial compensation for their transportation costs.

Procedure

A modified, placebo-controlled, cross-over design, based on those used by Tirosh, Sadeh, Munvez, and Lavie (1993) and by Barkley, McMurray, Edelbrock, and Robbins (1990) was employed. Participants were assigned either to group one which followed a placebo-drug sequence or to group two which followed a drug-placebo sequence. There were five subjects in group one and six in group two. Subjects were randomly assigned to one of these two groups by the Pharmaceutical Department at the Royal University Hospital in Saskatoon. Only the Pharmaceutical Department had access to the order of conditions for each subject until the end of the trials. The stimulant medications and placebo pills were placed in colored capsules to prevent their identification. Pill distribution was under the surveillance and supervision of the developmental pediatrician on our research team. Dosages for both the stimulant medications and placebo pills were individualized with each subject remaining on his or her customary dosage as previously prescribed by his or her pediatrician. All children successfully completed the procedure without requiring the drug status to be identified.

One day prior to the onset of the study, all subjects were asked to refrain from taking their regular stimulant medication. After this washout period subjects underwent their first condition of either placebo pills or medication which lasted three days. A three day period was used for each condition as opposed to the seven to ten day period used in other studies (Barkley et al., 1990; Tirosh, Sadeh, Munvez, & Lavie, 1993) as the half-life of these drugs is less than 24 hours. In addition, several of the families felt that a seven day washout period would result in hardship to themselves and their child. On the third day of this condition subjects underwent testing at the Kinsmen Children's Center. The order of the administration of the vigilance and underlining tasks was counterbalanced to control for order effects due to fatigue and practice. Children were tested individually by an experimenter and parents completed questionnaires. Parents requesting the opportunity to observe the testing of their child or children did so through a one-way mirror.

All subjects wished to be tested on the weekend, to facilitate school attendance and parents' work schedules. Therefore, after the completion of the first testing session there were three days until the washout day for the second condition. Subjects were instructed to return to their regular medication for these three days. After the first condition another washout day was implemented followed by a second three day condition of either stimulant medication of placebo pills respectively. All participants then underwent a final testing session on the third day of this condition and their parents completed a second questionnaire. No subjects were exempt from the study on the basis of non-compliance which was defined as one entire day of failure to take the stimulant medication or placebo pills. See Table 1 for details about the subjects and their medications.

TABLE 1. Subject's ages, weights, and medication information.

Subject	Age	Weight (kgs)	Meds/dosage/time
1	12–10	38.2	Methylphenidate 20 mgs a.m. & noon
2	6–5	18.2	Methylphenidate 5.0 mgs a.m. & noon
3	7–4	19.4	Methylphenidate 10 mgs a.m. & 5.0 mgs noon
4	8–5	23.2	Methylphenidate 10 mgs a.m. & 5.0 mgs noon
5	9–0	22.0	Dexedrine 5.0 mgs a.m. & noon
6	13–8	47.1	Methylphenidate 20 mgs a.m. & noon
7	16–9	31.0	Methylphenidate S-R 40 mgs a.m.
8	9–8	28.3	Pemoline 56.25 mgs a.m.
9	9–11	32.1	Methylphenidate S-R 20 mgs a.m.
10	8–1	14.9	Pemoline 37.5 mgs a.m.
11	8–6	28.7	Methylphenidate 10 mgs a.m. & noon

Measures

Attention

We assessed attention using a vigilance task that was a shortened version of the task used by Nanson and Hiscock (1990) and Streissguth and colleagues (1984). This task was chosen rather than the more conventional forms of the vigilance task that use letter sequences because it was designed for younger children. In addition, this task has been shown to be sensitive to the effects of prenatal alcohol exposure on the performance of young children (Streissguth et al., 1984). Administration conditions were identical to those used by Nanson and Hiscock (1990) but the last block of trials was dropped as this block was shown to be difficult for all children. Total task time was then nine minutes as opposed to 12 minutes in the original study. This is comparable to the 10 minute task used by Aman and colleagues (1993).

The two dependent measures of this task were reaction time and errors of omission. The equipment used did not permit collection of errors of commission, usually the most sensitive measure of alcohol effects. Reaction time was defined as the elapsed time from the first screen fill with the critical stimuli to the time when the child depressed the mouse button. Errors of omission were defined as failure to respond to stimuli. The vigilance task was administered using a Macintosh (Apple) microcomputer.

Impulsivity

Impulsivity was assessed using a short form of the Underlining Test (Rourke, Bakker, Fisk, & Strang, 1983). Four of the thirteen possible subsets of this test were employed in this study. In each subset the child was required to underline the designated stimulus which appeared in a random sequence among a series of other similar stimuli. Subjects completed a practice sheet, untimed, prior to the commencement of each subset, which consisted of three lines of stimuli. Any errors made during practice with respect to the identification of stimuli were pointed out immediately and the practice trial was repeated.

In the first subset the child was required to underline a Greek cross each time it appeared in random sequence among a series of 235 geometric forms which included squares, stars, circles, triangles, and so forth. In the second subset, the participant was instructed to underline a nonsense letter which was interspersed in a random sequence of 126 letters. In the third subset, the figure to be identified was a diamond containing a square which in turn contained a diamond. This stimuli was interspersed among 168 similar figures in a random sequence. In the final subset subjects were required to underline the letter "s" which was interspersed among 360 randomized letters. Subsets two and three were identified by Rourke and colleagues (1983) as being significantly more difficult than one and four.

Subjects were given a standard set of instructions in which only the name of the stimuli varied for each subset. The scoring of this task, which was the number of correctly underlined stimuli minus the number of incorrectly underlined stimuli, provided a measure of impulsivity.

Hyperactivity

Although DSM-IV places hyperactivity and impulsivity on one dimension, we chose to measure hyperactivity separately, using a parent rating scale, the Abbreviated Symptom Questionnaire-Parents (ASQ-P; Conners, 1992). We would have preferred to obtain teacher rating scales as well, however the children attended several different school systems, each with different procedures for obtaining research data which made data collection too cumbersome. The ASQ-P is a checklist of symptoms and uses a four-point Likert-type scale for each. Normative scores are available for the child's age and sex.

On the third day of each of the two, three day conditions, one parent/guardian of each of the participants was asked to complete an ASQ-P. The parent/guardian was instructed to answer the questions based on their child or children's behavior in the past three days. If the parent/guardian indicated that their child or children's behavior was vastly different on day one than on day three, the parent/guardian was instructed to answer the questions based on the behavior observed on day three. It was asked that the same parent/guardian be responsible for completing both of the question-naires for each child.

Results

The vigilance and underlining tasks were scored according to the standard instructions provided for each task. Only nine of the 11 children completed the vigilance task, due to an equipment malfunction (see Tables 2 and 3).

For the vigilance task, a mean score for each of the three blocks was calculated for both the reaction time and errors of omission for each subject. Similarly, for the underlining test a mean score was calculated for each of the four subsets of the test for each subject. This was done to investigate whether subjects performance on the more difficult subsets (two and three) declined to a greater extent during the placebo than during the drug condition.

For the ASQ-P, T-scores (mean = 50, s. d. = 10) were calculated, based on the child's age and sex (see Figure 1).

Analyses of Variance (ANOVAs) with repeated measures were employed in the data analysis of the two tasks and the ASQ-P. In all analyses Time refers to the first or second time in which subjects were tested and group refers the subjects' random assignment to group one (placebo-drug) or group two (drug-placebo). A three-way

TABLE 2. Mean Reaction Times and Numbers of Errors on Vigilance Task.

| Subject | Reaction Time | | | | Errors | | | |
| | Placebo | | Drug | | Placebo | | Drug | |
	Mean	(s.d.)	Mean	(s.d.)	Mean	(s.d.)	Mean	(s.d.)
1	31.03	(1.94)	26.37	(2.35)	0.00	(0.00)	0.67	(0.58)
2	35.10	(34.52)	51.17	(3.04)	8.33	(1.53)	4.00	(1.00)
3	*	*	*	*	10.00	(0.00)	10.00	(0.00)
4	45.57	(18.01)	32.87	(2.69)	6.67	(2.52)	6.67	(1.15)
5	32.27	(7.07)	21.93	(5.28)	1.67	(2.08)	7.00	(1.00)
6	11.33	(19.63)	44.67	(40.81)	9.33	(1.15)	9.33	(0.58)
7	33.47	(4.44)	39.17	(4.62)	5.33	(0.58)	1.00	(1.00)
8	23.47	(2.23)	28.33	(1.42)	1.33	(0.58)	3.67	(2.08)
9	22.63	(0.31)	20.40	(1.15)	0.00	(0.00)	1.00	(1.00)
Mean	29.36	(10.21)	33.11	(11.03)	4.74	(4.01)	4.82	(3.60)

*No valid response for subject 3, so no reaction time existed.

(Time × Group × Block) ANOVA with repeated measures for the vigilance task and a three-way (Time × Group × Subset) ANOVA with repeated measures for underlining test were conducted to compare subjects' performance on each of these tasks during placebo and medication conditions within and between groups. To determine whether the parents' observations of the children's hyperactivity on the ASQ-P differed between the placebo and medication conditions, within and across groups a two-way (Time × Group) ANOVA with repeated measures was carried out. Finally, Pearson Product Moment correlation coefficients were calculated between the scores for each of the vigilance and underlining tasks and the ASP-Q scores to investigate the correspondence between the subjects' performance on each of the two tasks and the parents observations of the subjects' hyperactivity. The overall means for all subjects during the placebo condition and during the drug condition for each task were calculated and used in the correlation.

Contrary to prediction there were no significant effects for the vigilance or underlining tasks for any measure. In addition none of the correlations between experimental measures and the parents' observations were significant.

However, the ASQ-P scores were significantly lower for drug (mean 68. 36, s.d. 17.4) vs. placebo (mean 84.4, s.d. 14.0) conditions ($F = 8.66$; $p = 0.016$). The children's mean hyperactivity scores were two standard deviations lower on medication than on placebo.

TABLE 3. Mean numbers of hits on an Underlining Task

Subject	Placebo		Drug	
	Mean	(s.d.)	Mean	(s.d.)
1	15.25	(11.70)	17.50	(8.81)
2	5.75	(4.92)	5.75	(2.87)
3	10.75	(2.06)	8.75	(3.77)
4	7.00	(7.87)	15.25	(9.91)
5	10.25	(7.89)	13.50	(13.30)
6	9.25	(2.50)	10.25	(3.30)
7	19.25	(13.60)	18.00	(12.30)
8	0.25	(10.40)	-1.50	(5.20)
9	15.00	(4.24)	9.50	(10.08)
10	21.00	(14.47)	24.25	(13.10)
11	16.75	(8.66)	13.25	(9.91)
Mean	11.86	(6.24)	12.22	(6.86)

Discussion

To the best of our knowledge, this is the first study to investigate the efficacy of stimulant medication in children with ADHD and FAS. This study provides mixed support for the effectiveness of stimulants in the treatment of ADHD and ADD in children with FAS.

In the present sample, stimulant medications did not significantly improve sustained attention by reducing the time required to respond to a stimulus or by reducing the number of stimuli that went unnoticed. This is in marked contrast to other studies showing treatment effects for children with pure ADHD (Abikoff & Gittelman, 1985; Pelham et al., 1990) and for children with developmental disorders (Aman et al., 1991; Dickerson-Mayes, Crites, Bixler, Humphrey, & Mattison, 1994). However, the significant effect of stimulant medications on the parent rating scales suggests that the children's hyperactivity might have been reduced even if the effects were not evident on the experimental tasks. In addition, the scores for all the experimental tasks and the parent ratings showed a great deal of variability, suggesting that the children's responses were highly idiosyncratic. This points to the need in clinical practice to titrate individual children's dosages carefully and monitor them closely.

It is possible that hyperactivity is the only domain of ADHD in children with FAS that is affected by stimulant medications. In this study, parents had a three day interval in which to monitor the

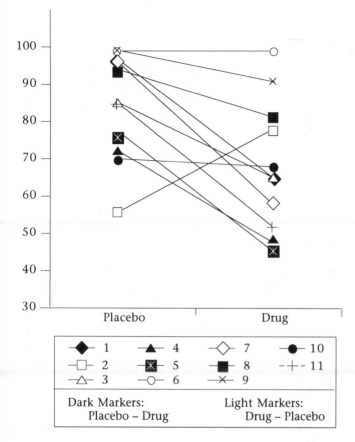

Figure 1. Individual subjects' ASQ-P t-scores.

children's behavior. Therefore their ratings were based on a much larger sample of behavior than is typically used in a clinical setting. Thus it is not surprising that parents were able to detect treatment effects that were not sampled by the experimental tasks.

It is the parents and teachers of children with FAS who bring the children to the attention of clinicians because of their disruptive behavior. It is the responsibility of parents, and sometimes teachers, to administer the medication and monitor its effectiveness in real-life settings. Thus a treatment that is salient to parents in reducing a difficult behavior may be sufficient to justify its use, even if it fails to produce as great a treatment effect as it does with other groups of children with ADHD, as medications appear to have been in this study.

There are several limitations of the present study that may have reduced its ability to detect any effects of the medication on the children's behavior directly.

First, all our subjects had a prior history of successful treatment with stimulant medication, so that they were a subgroup of all children with FAS known to be responsive to stimulants. This group of stimulant-responsive subjects is sometimes referred to as "pure" hyperactive children (Swanson, Barlow, & Kinsbourne, 1981). Not all children with FAS may fall into this pure hyperactive group, and the medication responses of children who are not pure hyperactives may be quite different from those in our study.

Second, our sample size was small, which compounded the problems of generalizability due to subjects' different ages, weights, dosages, types of preparations (long-acting or short-acting), and times of testing (four subjects were administered medications once per day, and six were administered medications twice per day). The small sample size also limited our statistical power. With a sample of this size only large effects could be detected. Further research involving larger samples of children are needed. Expanding the sample to include children with Fetal Alcohol Effects (FAE) would have increased the potential subject pool, but at the expense of having a less well defined sample.

Third, our experimental tasks lacked standardized scores based on age. Given the wide age range and developmental levels of the children involved, it is possible that age-corrected scores would have been more sensitive to treatment effects than were the experimental tasks. The effects due to age may have been greater than the treatment effects thus masking the latter. In addition, the experimental tasks were very difficult for some of the more severely handicapped children, and one could not complete the vigilance task.

Further research using less demanding tasks, narrower age and weight ranges, and more controlled dosages is needed as treatment effects may vary according to these variables.

In a clinical setting, individual calibration of dosage and type of medication is critical. In our clinical practice, we find that individual children often show idiosyncratic reactions to medication, and a period of trial and errors is needed to establish a personalized treatment regime. Good communication between the family, the school, and the physician is critical to the success of the treatment plan. Parents do appear to be able to detect treatment effects and are able to monitor their children's treatment effectively. In addition, stimulant medication is only one component of a treatment program for children with FAS and ADHD, and should be used after behavior modification and parent counseling have been well established. Medication is a useful adjunct and may increase the effectiveness of other treatments, but in our experience is seldom useful when used alone. Finally, stimulant medications may be mis-used and should never be prescribed for a family where issues of parental substance abuse and other forms of severe family psychopathology are present. However, in carefully chosen cases, stimulant medications may be a useful addition to a multidisciplinary treatment program for families of children with FAS.

A Demonstration Classroom
for Young Children with FAS

Patricia Tanner-Halverson

In 1990, a two-year grant from the Arizona State Department of Education was awarded to develop a Special Education pilot program, which was continued for an additional two years after the end of the initial grant period. The goal of this four-year project was to identify appropriate management and educational techniques for children prenatally exposed to alcohol. We began with a collection of techniques gathered from both the Fetal Alcohol Syndrome and Attention Deficit Disorders literatures (Gold & Sherry, 1984; Shaywitz, Cohen, & Shaywitz, 1980; Stokes & Osnes, 1986; Streissguth, Barr et al. 1986; Streissguth, LaDue, & Randels, 1986; Streissguth & Randels, 1988) and added methods as the years progressed. Many educational strategies were field tested, and in some cases modified, for maximum effectiveness with children prenatally exposed to alcohol.

The class initially comprised seven boys prenatally exposed to alcohol, from a pool of twelve identified children six to nine years old, who exhibited the slowest academic gains and the most disruptive behavior. Children were examined by a dysmorphologist at a clinic sponsored by the Indian Health Service. By the end of the initial two years, two boys were added to total nine boys in the class, all low-average to average intelligence, as measured by the WISC-III.

At the end of the first two years, all nine boys demonstrated marked behavioral improvements and modest academic gains. Although three children were being seriously considered for residential placement prior to placement in the program, all of them remained in the district. In addition, the project enabled the district to remove the highly disruptive students from the regular classrooms until their behavior was more manageable, thereby lessening the impact of their disruptive behavior on the general school population. Towards the end of the project's first year, students began gradual mainstreaming into regular classes with few behavioral difficulties.

An important outcome of the project was the development of effective methods and strategies to teach and maximize learning in children prenatally exposed to alcohol. Five key concepts were identified: structure (Streissguth, LaDue, & Randels, 1986), consistency, brief presentations, variety and repetition. This chapter describes some of the specific methods and strategies we found to be beneficial.

Environmental Strategies

Using well-defined areas and images aids memory and satisfies a child's need for structure. It decreases the disorganization of the neurologically impaired child and increases the child's sense of control. For example, use a specific shape and color to define an area. Stamp a red triangle on math items, or a blue circle on reading items. Label work centers and other locations with signs that have both the words and the pictures that denote the specific activities that take place at each location. Use pictorial cues as reminders of class routines. For example, use stick figures to denote actions. Make pictorial signs for special room areas and locations.

A "brain map," or "memory map," is a one-page pictoral description of a lesson. These maps enhance a child's ability to think in terms of graphic relationships and help establish lasting connections. Ask students to construct their own maps. In the process of creating memory maps, they are drawing pictures in their brains that will last much longer than will words.

Limit the number of objects and displays visible in the room at one time and try to avoid the use of mobiles. When a visual display, such as a bulletin board, is not in use remove it or keep it covered with a piece of light blue-gray flannel. Keep work areas clean except for the materials being used. Similarly, keep worksheets uncluttered and leave a lot of white space on the page; instead of having 25 pictures on one sheet, have only five.

Use preferential seating. Seat the child with FAS up front, next to the teacher. Parents state that eye contact may need to be maintained when speaking with children prenatally exposed to alcohol, or they often do not "hear" the person speaking to them. In groups, seat the child directly across from the teacher, looking directly at the teacher, so that eye contact can be maintained continually. This engages both auditory and visual channels. If the child sits beside the instructor, eye contact cannot be maintained continually.

Transitions

Children with FAS have trouble with activity changes and with keeping track of the beginning, middle and end of activities. If a child can not finish an assignment within the allotted time period, he/she will not feel the sense of completion that comes with finishing a task, thereby making changing to a new task problematic. Adapt tasks and materials to minimize frustration. Shorten the time of the task and the number of problems to be worked, and simplify material and concepts. Work towards a sense of completion. Breaking work into small pieces will reduce anxiety and decrease the child's tendency to think "I will never get this all done."

Try to draw a picture of time. For example, use a clear plastic cup or an hour glass timer so both time elapsed and time remaining in a session can be seen. Make paper chains, with the chain's links representing a specific period of time, and tear off a link as each time period passes. Alert children in advance of an activity change with an early warning system. "We have ten more minutes to finish up . . . five more minutes to finish up . . . You should be finishing up!"

Teaching Organizational Skills

Ask parents to get children ready for the next day by getting school materials and the next day's clothing laid out and organized the night before.

Give direct instruction about and emphasize thinking skills. Ask the student, "How did you figure that out? What did you do first?" Teachers and parents should model this process by thinking out loud so that the student hears the adult's thinking processes and strategies.

At the beginning of each day, review with the child the activities of the day before and identify the primary goal(s) for the current day. This is also a good time to comment on any successes, even small ones, of the day before.

Keep tasks short.

Give explicit, limited, concrete, brief and carefully defined directions.

Avoid expressions such as "Does that ring a bell?" or "The cat got your tongue?" or "Let's talk turkey." These expressions are very confusing to children who are concrete thinkers. We have found that phrases that can not be translated literally cause confusion, often identified by a quizzical look on the child's face.

Increasing Attention

Use eye contact, or touch, or call a child by name before giving directions. Make sure, first, that the child is listening by engaging him/her. Move closer to the child. Break down instructions into very small pieces and do not assume that a child has the prerequisite knowledge necessary for an assignment. A child may have the prerequisite knowledge on Monday, lack it on Tuesday and Wednesday, and then have it again on Thursday. Give additional anticipatory explanations. Cover the contingency cases, the "What If's . . . ?"

A tape recorder helps with memory problems, because it allows the child to listen to information repeatedly. This reinforces learning. Ear phones, with no sound coming through them, block out extraneous noise and can increase attention when a child is recording material and playing it back.

Use a study carrel as a privilege. Call the carrel "The Office" and decorate it like an "office." Never place a child in this quiet area as punishment.

A lesson outline at the beginning of an exercise increases listening comprehension. For reading exercises, for example, an outline clarifies the organization of a story. Prepare a child for a listening or reading exercise by talking first about what to look for in the story. Ask a child to repeat back directions in his/her own words so that you can be certain that the child has processed and understands the information. Spend time on describing or comparing objects, events and details of a story to increase the child's awareness of details often missed because of short attention spans. For example, "Tell me everything you can about the dog . . . what is his color, describe his ears and coat, his personality, who are his friends and enemies?" Sustained attention is a skill that can be gradually increased over a period of time. Create a chart that graphs the child's progress with sustained attention. Allow the child to make it himself/herself.

Employ random participation in the classroom (especially in reading groups) to limit a child's ability to predict when she may be called on to participate. This process creates a dynamic tension in addition to increased attention among students. For instance, a child will think, "The teacher may call on me next so I'd better be ready."

Use pictures, objects, facial expressions and kinesthetics to maintain attention. It is difficult to maintain attention when information is presented through voice alone. Information needs to be presented visually and kinesthetically to supplement auditory presentations whenever possible. Teach adjectives and adverbs by using the senses. For example, ask a child to feel the difference between hot and cold. Begin with concrete adjectives and adverbs that can be demonstrated via tactile or kinesthetic means or via comparison of concrete objects. For example, compare big-little, loud-soft, and high-low.

When working with a group at a table, use a "privacy board" constructed from a piece of heavy cardboard, folded into thirds, to visually delineate each child's work area and to block out visual stimulation from other children's work. Cut the shield down so that the child can see other student faces, but not the table.

Controlling Impulsivity

There is nothing wrong with being fast and right, but the impulsive or hyperactive child is usually fast and wrong. They try a fast guess, fail to process information and act without thinking.

We find that many children lack or have compromised "executive functioning skills." Executive functioning skills are those skills which enable us to decide that we want something, consider different choices about how to obtain the desired object, initiate and sustain a complex sequence of actions to obtain the object, and self-monitor and self-correct if the chosen plan of action is not working. Children affected by FAS respond immediately to impulses, without the "in-between" part that enables rule-governed behavior.

Understanding this deficit is important when dealing with behaviors that could lead to danger if impulses are not controlled or thought about. Children must be taught appropriate "habits" for these behaviors. Habit is behavior that is impulse-response, without the critical thinking in-between.

Give complete directions before handing out materials. Fold test booklets or sheets in half, and staple them shut so children cannot start the test until a pre-arranged hand signal is given, or bell is rung. Give this signal at the end of the direction and question period. Provide self-checking materials that require a child to search for mistakes and correct his/her work before turning it in to the teacher. Require that children defend their answers. Do not be satisfied with factual answers only. What is the reasoning behind the answer? Require explanations about how conclusions were reached as part of the answer.

It is difficult for neurologically impaired children to wait for their turn because they respond to thoughts (impulses) with action. They also may have difficulty grasping temporal relationships. To help a child understand when it is his/her turn, take a small toy (such as a three-inch teddy bear), and say, "Here is the rule. When the bear is in your hand, it is your turn." When a child responds out of turn, instead of any negative response, we can politely ask, "Is the bear in your hand?"

Discipline

Be firm but supportive. Consistently adhere to rules. Make sure the rules are clearly understood. Adherence to rules should have pre-established positive consequences; rule-breaking should have pre-established negative consequences. Avoid intimidation and humiliation. When correcting a child, speak softly, close to his or her ear (unless the child is tactually defensive). Try giving a look that says "I saw what you did." Recognize their response to this look with another look that says "I see that you saw." Use positive statements to tell children where their place is ("This is your desk, this is where you are supposed to be") instead of using negatives ("You are not supposed to be away from your desk").

Do not debate or argue about the rules. This is not the great debate. Make the "broken record" technique a key method of communication. Using a broken record means that the teacher or parent uses the identical words repeatedly. Say only, "Just do it," each time. You can negotiate or debate about the usefulness of a rule, but not after a rule has just been broken.

Behavior modification techniques, especially positive reinforcement, will work at times with some children. Track virtues and sainthood. For example, each time a child initially takes the time to think before responding to a comment, note the positive behavior by saying, "Excuse me, I need to make a note of this." Then make an X on a card that tracks successful inhibition of responses.

Use negative reinforcement (the removal of a reward) rather than outright punishment to respond to minor offenses. For example, if a child is always out of his/her seat, at the nurse's office, or in the bathroom, try the following. Wait until the child has left his/her seat and then announce to the class, "Everyone who is sitting in their assigned seat right now will get a special treat." If the child is out of the room, time it so that he/she returns while you are distributing the treat.

Survey the children to determine which reinforcements are interesting and valuable to them. Prepare a list, or better yet, make "my choice" cards, from which the child may choose an activity or prize. To make "my choice" cards for students, list and draw pictures of individual activities the children find reinforcing on small pieces of cardboard (two by three inches), punch a hole in each card and put the cards on a ring. When it is time for a reward, students can choose the activity they desire from the cards. School activities to use for reinforcement may include being the line leader, being the aide for the day, being a hall monitor for a week, or applying a washable tattoo. Distinguish rewards to be done with an adult or with someone else from those that can be done alone.

Reduce lag time by giving enough activities to maintain productivity. Keep the child busy so there is no opportunity to become distracted. Structure the environment so that there is little or no opportunity for off-task behavior.

Specifically label obnoxious behavior. "When you scream at me like you are doing right now or shove against me to get out of the elevator first, that is really obnoxious."

Use the concept of a "peace chair" or "time-in" rather than "time out." We isolate a child to take away the classroom cheering section. When his/her peers are not around he/she does not have to save face.

Consult with families to help at home with behavior management. Teach them these techniques.

Dealing with Hyperactivity

Limit the type and number of new situations encountered at one time. Children with FAS become easily overwhelmed and overstimulated, resulting in misbehavior such as temper tantrums or shutting down completely. Gaze aversion may signal overstimulation. Children may turn their entire body away or even move their desk off to the side. They are not necessarily being belligerent. They just may be trying to get the stimulation under control.

Anticipate and know danger signs and situations. Build relaxation time into the program. Try using soft background music on the radio to calm a child. When Mary starts tapping her feet and drumming her fingers, she needs to discharge that energy or she might erupt into aggressive behavior. Try sending her to deliver a note to the office or another teacher, having her take a little break, or speed walking around the playground until she feels calmer.

Medication may need to be considered. Keep an open mind about medications and give recommendations for trials on medication a fair chance. Some of our children showed marked improvement in their behavior and ability to attend and learn after they were put on medication. If the child is on medication, it is better to start the day with medication, if the behavior warrants it, than to chase the behavior once it is out of control.

Provide lessons that emphasize manual or physical expression. Ask children to draw the activity being discussed or fill in design sheets with color while the instructor is teaching. Avoid long periods of desk work and do not keep a child in during recess. Give additional short breaks during the day. Provide regularly scheduled walks and other physical activities.

Protect the child from over stimulation. Control television watching and avoid video games, such as Nintendo. Nintendo-style games will overstimulate most children with FAS very quickly. If a child cannot handle all the excitement of the circus, a carnival or a pow-wow, do not go or shorten the time in attendance.

Have a respite plan in place for when a child becomes overwhelmed. Initially the teacher should direct the child to use the respite plan when appropriate. Ultimately the child will learn what he/she can do when he/she starts to feel overwhelmed and will remove himself/herself, with a pre-arranged signal to the teacher. For example, the child may be allowed to leave the classroom and go for a walk with the counselor or assistant principal, or go to the nurse, lie down, and visualize fishing in a quiet, peaceful stream.

Self Esteem

Recognize successes each day. Say good-bye to every student at the end of every day with an upbeat statement. Recognize some accomplishment or good behavior during that day.

You are a powerful model for appropriate behavior. Try a coping model rather than a mastery model. When the instructor models a behavior perfectly, children may just shut down, perhaps because they feel they can never do it perfectly. Model the problem the child is having and then model the solution or a strategy in slow, easy or partial steps.

Make sure you are testing knowledge not attention span. Avoid timed tests, make the test short, and perhaps give the test individually. Keep a careful watch on students to make sure they are working and not staring out the window.

Provide positive incentives for finishing. Instead of focusing on children who do not finish, pay attention and reward those who do. Recognize the child for partially correct responses. "Yes, the answer is wrong, but look, you did this part right."

Avoid asking "why" questions. Use "how," "who," "what" and "where" instead. Asking "why" often places the child in a defensive mode. These children often finds themselves on the defensive. Do not add to the burden.

Memory

Take three forks and three napkins when you go through the lunch line, so that when the child with memory problems forgets his/her utensils you are ready. Repeat and restructure continually. Express ideas in different ways and use different modalities. For example, tell a short story and ask the children to close their eyes and picture the scene in their minds. Ask children to write ideas, visualize them, hear them, act them out.

Reading

The easiest way to learn to read and write is to work on a vertical plane, not a horizontal plane. Get an old music stand and put the book on it. Lying flat on the floor to read moves the material to the vertical plane. Rewrite text directions at a lower reading level. Use a highlighter to emphasize and identify key or important words in a reading passage. Outline letters with glue for a three-dimensional boundary or use three-dimensional plastic or foam letters, numbers and shapes. Use pipe cleaners to make letters or numbers.

Children with FAS may have figure-ground or foreground-background confusion. Use a black board if one is available as it gives better contrast than does a green board. Using tapes and listening centers helps with auditory figure-ground problems, such as distinguishing a voice from competing sounds. Read a passage with the same word repeated. Have the child hold up their hand every time they hear the word.

For visual figure-ground exercises draw an outline of a figure that overlaps with another one. Ask the child to trace the outlines with his/her finger. Start with two simple figures overlapping slightly and proceed in gradual steps to several figures overlapping. Use "hidden picture" puzzles and color-by-number pictures.

Avoid phonics to teach reading, unless you are certain auditory processing skills are adequate. Phonics requires analysis and synthesis, skills that many neurologically impaired children do not have. Educators may also have difficulty using a phonics approach to teach reading to children with FAS because of the children's limited ability to generalize. Children may have difficulty integrating parts into a whole, generalizing from the specific to the universal and seeing how universals relate to specifics.

For children who have difficulty with directionality (reading from left to right), using colored dots to represent left and right might help. Use a green "go" dot on the left side of the line and a red "stop" dot on the right. Always start on the "go" and end on the "stop." Carefully observe eyes while a child is reading to determine eye movement for "regressive" eye movements and vertical shifts. This may be an essential part of a child's directional and/or lateral perception difficulty.

The use of a city map to play a directional game may be helpful. Ask the child to start at a specified point and direct him/her to another part of town. "Turn left, then go two blocks, then turn right." Place a small lavender "L" on back of the left hand and a red "R" on the right hand, thereby creating a continually available clue identifying left from right. Use color coding according to position in a word, for example, the first letter or group of letters in a word is always green, the middle is yellow and the end is red.

Math

Work on the concept of the number, not just rote counting. "How many of these make four? Which number is bigger, four or two? Look at your fingers. Which is more?" Spend extra time on money concepts and making change. Children with FAS have a lot of trouble dealing with the abstraction of money. Use actual coins in teaching money concepts. Play "Restaurant" or "Shopping." Bring menus and set up a restaurant or store with real items. Provide practice of addition and subtraction with a computer that gives immediate feedback to the child. Provide practice with money problems using a computer software program. Computer games are motivating and fun for children.

Avoid mixing addition and subtraction problems. Put math problems of the same process on a single sheet of paper or on a single line. Make operation symbols extra large, bolded or color-coded. If children do not want to do simple adding and subtracting again because "that is baby stuff," give them another sheet that looks complex, but is still simple.

General Strategies

When teaching a lesson, do not assume that children will generalize the information to new situations. They probably will not. We have to point out other situations and get them to actively think about it. "When else would you do this? Do you think it would work here? How is that situation similar to this one?" You must also help link new learning to prior experience.

Help children to appreciate the value of failure. Mistakes show us what does not work. Mistakes are windows of discovery. Children with learning problems should aim for success not perfection. Children can control the size of their mistakes by taking the time to think about the consequences of what they do. What is important is not that we never make mistakes, but that we learn from those mistakes. Share some of your amusing mistakes. Stop at key points in order to determine the child's understanding and then go on to the next point.

Encourage children to develop a success orientation. Focus on successes not failures. Take it in small pieces and count each success. Catch them being good, doing things right. Notice it! Mark charts you have made when children do things correctly, not when children do things incorrectly.

Summary

We found that children prenatally exposed to alcohol responded very well to these strategies. However, when they were re-introduced on a full-time or nearly full-time basis to the mainstream environment, difficulties often arose. Their hyperactivity frequently escalated with the increased environmental stimulation. They were especially sensitive to the haptic activity (body movement) of 15 or more students maneuvering around them. A few students compensated for this by staying on the fringes of unstructured group activity, but this was difficult in a crowded classroom. Using a study carrel and earphones became critical to maintaining productivity.

The students who participated in this project are now in junior high or high school. We no longer see the low self-esteem and rage we observed initially. They are more aware and accepting of their limitations. Developing alternative, self-enhancing, pro-social ways to deal with some of their frustrations has been encouraging. We have discovered that a highly structured, consistent, repetitive program gives these children a cocoon of safety from which to explore their world.

A National Survey of State Directors of Special Education Concerning Students with FAS

Thomas Wentz

Maternal alcohol use during pregnancy can cause birth defects and chronic maternal alcoholism can result in Fetal Alcohol Syndrome (FAS) (Coles, Smith, Fernhoff, & Falek, 1985; Ernhart et al., 1987; Graham, Hanson, Darby, Barr, & Streissguth, 1988; Jones & Smith, 1973; Jones, Smith, Ulleland, & Streissguth, 1973; Lemoine, Harousseau, Borteyru, & Menuet, 1968). FAS has been recognized as the leading identifiable cause of mental retardation in the United States for the past ten years (Abel & Sokol, 1986). In addition to maternal alcoholism, binge and social drinking may cause a wide range of problems, including developmental delays, learning disabilities, behavioral and emotional problems, attention deficits, and hyperactivity (Streissguth, Bookstein, Sampson, & Barr, 1993). The wide range of deficits incurred as consequences of the known levels of maternal consumption of alcohol during pregnancy may impact far greater numbers of children in our schools.

This chapter briefly presents the results of a survey of state directors of special education, completed in 1995. The purpose of this survey was to identify answers to the questions of school information on Fetal Alcohol Syndrome in each of the fifty states. The survey consisted of a two-page pamphlet of 41 factual and opinion questions and a third page of three open-ended questions. State directors of special education or their designees from all 50 states' departments of public instruction were surveyed. All fifty states responded to the survey.

School Populations

No state counted the number of its students with Fetal Alcohol Syndrome (K-12) for Special Education purposes or for any other educational purposes. No educational census of the Fetal Alcohol Syndrome student (K-12) population is presently available in the United States.

FAS prevalence research nationwide is inconclusive. Four states (South Carolina, Washington, New York, and North Dakota) have completed statewide FAS prevalence studies while two other states (South Dakota and Alaska) were in the process of conducting such research. One state, North Dakota, has published these data (Burd & Martsolf, 1993).

Demographic data about students with FAS: This survey included an attempt to gather demographic information (income, race, and retention rates) by which to develop a FAS student profile. Regarding family income, one state collected data related to this category; the remaining 49 states reported not collecting income data. Regarding race, a number of states collected data on race for both regular and special education students, but not all states. However, no state collected data on race related specifically to students with FAS. Finally, data collection on retention rates was the same; no state collected data for students with FAS.

Services and Administration

Is FAS a recognized Special Education eligibility category for special educational services in your state? No state specifically serves the disability category of Fetal Alcohol Syndrome. Furthermore, none of the 50 states had plans to recognize Fetal Alcohol Syndrome as a disability category in the future. The reported obstacles to serving students with FAS included lack of information about FAS (76% of respondents), FAS is not a problem — societal denial regarding FAS (56%), lack of a clear federal mandate (53%), lack of other resources — lack of trained physicians (52%), and lack of funding (49%).

In your state's Department of Special Education, is there a designated FAS position? No state education agency (SEA) has an administrative FAS position. Alaska, which previously had a statewide FAS Coordinator in their Department of Public Instruction, lost the position due to recent funding cuts.

Are there any plans to add or include an FAS position? One state, Mississippi, had plans for adding a state-level FAS administrative position. The 49 remaining states did not have plans to add such an administrative position.

In your opinion, is there a need for such a position? Ten states responded positively ("yes") to this question. Three states claimed they wanted the expertise of a person trained in this area but not for this disability category alone. Two states were undecided at the moment the interview was conducted and two states did not respond to the question. Thirty-three states said there was not a need for such a position.

Educational costs of students with FAS. No state could identify the educational costs of serving Fetal Alcohol Syndrome students.

Identification

Numerous programs now exist to aid in the identification of handicapped children for the purpose of intervention. Child Find, Early Periodic Screening, Diagnosis, and Treatment (EPSDT) program, "At Risk" under Part H, and the Special Education referral and assessment process are specific examples of federally mandated programs to identify and intervene with handicapped students. Medical diagnosis and birth defects registries are two additional ways of identifying handicapped children.

How does your state identify FAS children? 13 states reported using medical diagnosis and two of the 13 states reported using a birth defects registry to identify students with FAS. Twenty-five states did not have a program or mechanism to specifically identify students with FAS. Six states reported no attempt at identifying FAS children.

Implementation of Individual Education Plan (IEP) Requirements

Of those FAS students on IEPs, what percentage participate in specific placements? No state could identify the number of students on IEPs with a diagnosis of FAS.

In your opinion, how effective or ineffective is inclusion for children with FAS? Forty-eight states had no data for this question. Two states felt that inclusion was very effective but had no supporting data.

Educational Interventions

Does your state subscribe to or endorse a specific program(s) of education or training for FAS students? Forty-seven states did not have a specific program of instruction for students with FAS. Three states utilized the *Fetal Alcohol and other Drug Effected* (FADE) program (Alaska, Oregon, and Washington) developed by the Western Regional Center, Portland, OR.

Although they did not report subscribing to or endorsing a specific program or training, three states did report having FAS-specific programming areas (California, Nevada, and New Mexico). Twenty-one states reported using nonspecific programming for students with FAS; in other words, programming was based upon existing Special Education programming or individual needs based upon the immediate presenting problem. Twelve states did not know what programming was provided for students with FAS. Six states said no programming was provided. Three states had no data to respond. One state leaves the responsibility for programming to the local educational agency (LEA). Two states did not complete the survey, and one state did not respond to the question.

The barriers reported that impede programming for students with FAS included lack of preservice preparation by universities and colleges (71%), lack of research on successful educational interventions (69%), lack of screening, assessment, and evaluation devices (65%), lack of available inservice programs (58%), and lack of federal and state mandates and financial support (45%).

Teacher Qualifications and Training

Does your state offer training (classes, seminars, inservices, etc.) for Special Educators about FAS students? Fifteen states reported having provided FAS training for special educators, and 13 of the same states provided FAS training for regular educators. The remaining 35 states either did not provide such inservice training or did not know if such training was available. No state required FAS inservice training for continuing certification.

Does your state offer training for Preservice Special Educators about FAS students? One state, New York, required both special and regular preservice educators to take an FAS specific class.

Severity of the Problem

How extensive is the FAS problem in your state? We organized the responses to this open-ended question into five categories:

(a) *Very extensive.* Eight state respondents indicated, quite strongly, that Fetal Alcohol Syndrome was a very extensive problem in their states.

(b) *Extensive.* Nine states saw the FAS problem as extensive or significant. However, many respondents were quick to point out they had no data to back up their claims.

(c) *Moderate, mild, a problem.* Seven states viewed the scope of the problem of fetal alcohol as moderate, mild, or a problem.

(d) *Not an extensive problem.* Two states felt FAS was not an issue of concern.

(e) *Do not know about the extent or it is not a focus.* Twenty-four states did not know the numbers of affected students and one state said FAS was not a focus of attention any longer.

What is the educational climate surrounding FAS in your state? Responses ranged from "yes, we are organized and we are responding at the state level with interagency collaboration," to responses and events that did not respond to the question. Again, responses generally could be organized into five categories:

(a) *Discussion and action.* The states of Alaska, Washington, Oregon, South Dakota, and Nevada are discussing FAS and education and acting on their discussions in varying degrees. Alaska, after having a statewide FAS coordinator, lost the position as a result of funding cuts by the legislature. However, it was the Alaska education agency that initiated the request to the Western Regional Center, Portland, Oregon, for a teacher preparation and student intervention program for FAS, that led to the development of the FADE program.

(b) *Discussion without action.* Approximately six states responded that discussion but no action was taking place regarding education and FAS/FAE in their states. Mississippi, Idaho, New York, West Virginia, Nebraska, and New Mexico could all be roughly classified under this area with some variation. A statement from one state is typical:

> "I think that FAS is being embraced as being a problem that special educators are going to have to learn more about and going to have to address . . . I think educationally we are becoming more aware of the problem with children who suffer from Fetal Alcohol Syndrome and ironically I think it is not only FAS making us more aware of FAS but it is also the problems with crack babies and those types of drug-related birth problems, FAS is in there with that whole thing . . ."

(d) *No discussion, do not know, or no specific response.* The 39 remaining states figured into this classification, based upon their generally similar responses, such as:

> "I am not familiar with that nomenclature [FAS]."
>
> "In special education there has been no conversation."
>
> "I do not hear much about it."
>
> "I think individually and probably more medically than anywhere else there is a great concern about it. It just has not hit the educational environment."
>
> "I do not even know if it exists."
>
> "The issue is prevention, rather than service. They are identified through the hospitals, they are identified through the Baby Net 0-2, and then they are served as

needed in the public schools and it is really not one of our big issues."

"I have been here for two years and the first time I heard of it was when I got your survey."

"This is Special Education. Are you sure you have the right office?"

What are the three greatest problems confronting state directors of special education regarding FAS/FAE? In thirteen states the greatest problem reported was lack of knowledge, information, awareness, or education. Seven states reported that the lack of procedures to identify children with FAS was the first, greatest problem. The most often reported second greatest problem was lack of resources and funding. Another often-reported area of concern was the lack of known successful educational interventions, service and administration, and teacher preparation programs for and about FAS/FAE students.

Conclusion and Recommendations

There exists a general lack of awareness about Fetal Alcohol Syndrome on the national level in Special Education. Awareness of FAS as an educational problem is very slow to emerge in public school education, specifically in Special Education. This survey collected the answers to questions about schools and the FAS student and was not intended to include a study of the reasons why Special Education is slow in recognizing this particular disorder. However, it is apparent from this study that the national emphasis of Special Education on de-categorization generally has presented an obstruction to prevalence estimates and to meeting of the educational needs of these students.

Awareness of a problem comes before funding and services, and services and interventions usually precede science-based interventions by 10 to 20 years. Therefore, the following actions are recommended:

1. Recognition of FAS as a disability category through federally mandated action to include formation of a national interagency task force to establish a research agenda and educational priorities.

2. Initiation of screening and identification procedures to determine the scope of the problem.

3. Development of preservice and inservice preparation programs to address the academic, behavioral, and emotional needs of FAS/FAE children.

4. Establishment of a national priority for the development of curriculum for the prevention of fetal alcohol and other drug affected infants for students grades 7-12.

Case Managers and Independent Living Instructors: Practical Hints and Suggestions for Adults with FAS

Claire Anita Schmucker

Perhaps an adult you know has been screened and diagnosed with FAS or FAE. Common characteristics of adults with FAS may include limited impulse control and anger management, minimal understanding of natural consequences, difficulties with financial management, limited ability to think in an abstract manner, problems generalizing from one situation to the next, problems in planning for the future (as the person with FAS lives primarily in the here and now), an ongoing need for immediate gratification, forgetfulness as a daily experience (for even the most routine and established task), a strict need for consistency, and on and on. Now what?

In addition to all of this, you also may find out that the person with FAS/FAE still is not eligible for services from the Division of Developmental Disabilities, at least at this time. This eliminates the provision of general case management, some state services for in-home care and assistance, and crisis intervention assistance. It dawns on you rather quickly that these things are now going to be the responsibility of you and your family, relatives, and friends. I began developing techniques for dealing with these issues as a private case manager to meet this need.

A good starting place is to understand fully that FAS is a diagnosable disability involving brain damage. The person who has been diagnosed with FAS is not going to recover instantly. He or she does not have a typical learning disability where some skills can be taught and maintained. And, most importantly, the person with FAS is most likely a lot more bothered by these problems than you are.

Because the characteristics that I first described are not going to miraculously "go away," you will need to adapt the environment this person lives in to accommodate his or her disabilities.

Guardianship and Housing

When possible, I start by recommending to the family that they obtain a guardian and/or a protective payee service. I also have found that if a family has the ability to set up a trust fund, this can be very helpful in providing future support.

Housing is a frequent concern especially for adults who continue to live with their parents or in rental properties. Perhaps the adult with FAS who continues to live with his/her family has brought home too many "friends" and you feel your family is not safe. Maybe the lack of anger control has offended all the neighbors in an apartment complex and, due to kicking in the front door, the person you know is being evicted. Can this person pool together resources to buy a small house, trailer, or condominium? Let the wall that gets punched in be his/her own. The person can have it fixed and do it all over again if he/she wants. Is the person eligible for public housing? Most public housing buildings have security entrances and an on-call manager.

If you are unable to facilitate the above changes, perhaps there are some smaller issues that you can take on.

Financial Management

A checking account can certainly be a major dilemma for a person with FAS. It is difficult enough for a person without FAS to manage money. Imagine how out of control it must feel for a person with FAS. The money is there — why not spend it? There are more checks — why not write them? The gal next door says that she really needs a new television — why not buy one for her? There is a sale at The Bon — I need new clothes. Before you know it, there is no money left and banking institutions that are willing to give "one more last chance" are limited.

One simple solution is to obtain a checking account that requires two signatures (and a bank which will actually adhere to the rule). Take each check and write "two signatures required" under the signature line. Make sure that the banks enter an "alert" onto this account. This will require them to check their computer for why the alert is on each time a transaction is completed. Your responsibility is to ensure that the alert status remains active. Make sure that the person is not issued an ATM card.

Once these logistics are taken care of, I try a variety of budget sheets with people to see what will work out best. A budget sheet can be as simple as a list of monthly bills that are due or as complex as listing all money spent. For my clients, the forms that tend to work best involve a self-reporting system. For example, divide up the monthly spending money and put a variety of amounts into individual boxes on the budget sheet. When there are no more boxes, there is no more money. These forms obviously should be individualized according to the person's monthly income.

If you are dealing with a payee service, try to arrange for spending money and grocery money to arrive on separate days. Have weekly spending money spread out as much as possible; even daily if this will be most beneficial to the person receiving the money. If you are involved with a trust fund, go into the bank and set up a plan for what the bank will do if the person arrives at the bank and demands their money. (What would happen to you if you went into the bank and demanded money?) It need not be a very complicated plan.

Credit and the intrusive solicitation that occurs for pre-approved credit is an ongoing issue for many people. I spend a lot of time canceling credit cards and orders that were placed over the phone. I also have tried to positively reinforce clients for not submitting credit applications and not purchasing things over the phone. For every uncompleted credit card application that gets turned over to you and not sent back in, perhaps as a reward there is a free movie rental, a new pair of earrings, a ride to work, or lunch at a restaurant.

Immediate Gratification/Impulse Control

Insisting that life is unfair and complaining that nothing ever gets accomplished is common among individuals with FAS. Within thirty minutes of buying a new car, I was asked by a client that I work with, "When are we going to get busy and get things done?" This affects many areas of the person's life and can result in financial fiascoes and illegal escapades.

Buy a camera and take pictures of all purchases and/or completed tasks, regardless of the importance to you. Put all the pictures in a scrapbook. I have seen scrapbooks with pictures varying from a new apartment to a new electric toothbrush to a picture of old cat hair (because that was the day that the cat was brushed). These scrapbooks can remind forgetful, impulsive clients of all they have accomplished.

Develop a system to track purchases and future requests. Have a notebook with pockets for each month so that each pocket has the advertisements for each item wanted that is affordable for that month. If it does not get purchased, it is not forgotten, just moved to the next pocket.

Inappropriate sexual behavior can also be discussed as an issue of impulse control. Sexual issues are raised frequently, and these issues should not be avoided. If the person you know or are working with is sexually active, it is a good idea to assist that person in having an HIV test on a regular basis. Discuss with the person that he/she could be an important asset to a health study and then sign him/her up at a local heath clinic. If accepted into a study, not only will the person receive free testing, but he or she may also be contacted about when to come in.

A client of mine found that he could call escort services in the yellow pages and not only did they accept checks and credit cards, they did more than escort you to dinner. "If it is illegal, Claire, then why are they listed in the Yellow Pages?" Good point. We ripped out those pages from his phone book.

Forgetfulness, Routine, and Generalization

Most of us learn quickly that if you do not water your plants, they die. The folks that I work with buy a lot of plants. Most pet owners know that we need to ensure that there is always water and food available. The folks that I work with often love animals, and I help them to use weekly feeder/water machines, and to post notes all over the house to remind them to keep the machines filled.

If someone is forgetting to turn off the oven or stove, unplug it and use a microwave. Or, start a tab for the person at a local restaurant and have them go there once a day for a hot meal and only keep cold meal items in the house.

Write things down for people and keep the rules simple. Have a list of things that have to be done that gets checked off daily or weekly. Put the list where it will be seen and call to remind the person that they should check the list.

Routine is extremely important and things can instantly go haywire with just the smallest change to the routine. A client with whom I work had a tab at a local restaurant. One day he discovered that the restaurant had closed down. It had taken him years to establish friendships there, learn the menu, learn how to drive there, remember what he could afford to order, and feel comfortable and enjoy going. The repercussions of this closure were amazing. It took me days to figure out what had upset him so much, and even longer to explain to him that perhaps his feelings over this change were related to why he wanted to quit his job and move. There was not one aspect of his life that was unaffected by this change.

Routines can be developed. Purchase season tickets (same seat each year) for sports events or theater shows. If a weekly routine is needed, perhaps signing up for a class at a local college would be helpful. Have the person take the same class semester after semester if they want. If a daily routine is needed, perhaps subscribe to the daily paper. Or perhaps a daily phone call at an expected time will be just enough to keep that person going. These are just ideas to spark your own creative solutions. Your plan needs to be realistic, and no matter how hard you have worked to set up the "perfect" routine, there is always the game that is canceled, the show that changes to a new day, or the fact that you are sick and unable to call at ten o'clock that morning.

For a person with FAS, not much will generalize from one situation to the next, so do not expect it to. Do not expect the person to remember what it is that you have developed for his or her benefit. What you should expect is to have to repeat what you have just discussed. And, if your intervention is not going to work because it will not generalize, change it! If you have told someone over and over to stay out of the street and he or she still goes into the street, perhaps your next option is to build a fence. If the neighbor has stopped taking advantage of your client, you may have to get ready to deal with the coworker who "only wants to borrow five dollars because he keeps forgetting his lunch."

Socialization

Unfortunately, these solutions are not going to address the ongoing isolation and loneliness with which so many adults with FAS are forced to deal. Developing friendships is next to impossible. Perhaps this is because your client is an adult who talks constantly about one subject, complains incessantly, is inappropriate (with interrupting and irrelevant comments), does not pick up on subtle (or direct) social cues, and is physically intrusive on others' personal space. Friendships tend to be mock situations created with paid providers.

A high rate of victimization seems to occur as a result of the ongoing pursuit for friendship by adults with FAS. If the other person is savvy enough, the abuse will persist. For example, a client bought a woman a television set because she "asked him to." She continued to ask for things until he had almost furnished her home, provided her with a summer wardrobe, and had let her boyfriend move in with him after the boyfriend had beaten him up.

Although there are not many direct preventive instructions that assist the adult with FAS in these situations, recognizing these characteristics can often be helpful in itself. Always keep your eyes open for situations that might arise.

Things we take for granted can be a major accomplishment in the life of a person with FAS. If you feel that you can assist such a person with attaining those accomplishments — great. The reality is that many family members and care providers have simply had enough. If arrangements can be made for others to assist in any small area, this will lighten the load of those already helping and free up more time for them to become the family and friends that are also needed.

An Advocacy Program for Mothers with FAS/FAE

Therese Grant, Cara Ernst, Ann Streissguth
and Jennifer Porter

Introduction

Pregnancy and childbirth among mothers who themselves have FAS/FAE is a topic that has not been adequately addressed, yet it is a problem with which clinicians who work with fetal alcohol affected patients are all too familiar. In this chapter, we review data from a recent study of this topic and describe an existing advocacy program that we believe is promising for working with these high-risk mothers during a critical time in their lives.

Mothers With Fetal Alcohol Syndrome and Fetal Alcohol Effects

Fetal Alcohol Syndrome (FAS) is a birth defect caused by heavy prenatal alcohol exposure. FAS is diagnosed when an individual has three characteristics: growth deficiency, a specific pattern of facial anomalies, and some manifestation of central nervous system (CNS) dysfunction. Individuals who have been prenatally exposed to alcohol, but who have only some of the characteristics of FAS may be diagnosed with Fetal Alcohol Effects (FAE) or Possible Fetal Alcohol Effects (PFAE) (Clarren & Smith, 1978). The CNS manifestations of FAS/FAE can be impaired intellectual ability; problems with learning, memory, attention, cognition, language, motor control, and others. Adolescents and adults with FAS/FAE often are described as having poor judgment, failing to consider consequences of their actions, being unresponsive to subtle social cues, and lacking reciprocal friendships.

In a recent study of 415 patients who previously had been diagnosed either FAS or FAE, 30 women were identified who had given birth (Streissguth, Barr, Kogan, & Bookstein, 1996). These 30 mothers

This paper was supported by the Center for Substance Absue Prevention, Public Health Service Grant # 4H86 SP02897, and the Stanley Foundation.

had a total of 55 children, and at the time of the research interview, over half of the women (54%) were not caring for all of their children. Thirty-six percent of the children had been removed from their mother's care by Children's Protective Services (CPS).

An alarming 40% of these FAS/FAE mothers (n=12) were drinking during at least one of their pregnancies (Table 1). Five mothers (17%) had a child who had been diagnosed FAS or FAE, and another four (13%) had children that the respondents suspected of being fetal alcohol affected. Table 1 illustrates other life history characteristics of these mothers that place them at high risk for dysfunctional parenting, including troubled childhoods, low IQ, low level of education, lack of income, and problems with the law.

Clearly, prenatal alcohol abuse by FAS/FAE mothers, and the subsequent delivery of alcohol-affected children, is a problem that demands attention. The magnitude of this problem is not insignificant when calculated against an FAS prevalence rate of one to three per thousand births (NIAAA, 1987) and an FAE prevalence rate several times higher. A cost-effective community solution is greatly needed. We believe the Seattle Advocacy model "Birth to 3" provides such a solution.

The Birth to 3 Advocacy Model

The Birth to 3 model began as a federally-funded research/demonstration project based upon the concept of paraprofessional advocacy (Grant, Ernst, McAuliff, & Streissguth, in press; Grant, Ernst, & Streissguth, in press; Grant, Streissguth, Phipps, & Gendler, 1996). It was developed to work with the highest risk mothers who abused alcohol and/or drugs during pregnancy and received little or no prenatal care. In brief, five paraprofessional advocates each work with a caseload of no more than 15 clients and their families from the birth of the target child until the child is three years old. The Birth to 3 model does not provide direct treatment or clinical services, but instead links women and their families with existing community resources. Advocates offer extensive practical assistance, guidance and a watchful eye.

There are no specific educational, occupational, or experiential requirements for the paraprofessional advocate positions. Advocates have the personal attributes of being good problem solvers, goal oriented, and empathic. They represent diverse ethnic backgrounds, most have worked in social service positions in the past, all have graduated from high school and have had some college education. They have experienced many of the same types of adverse life experi-

TABLE 1. Demographics of Birth to 3 mothers and mothers with FAS/FAE.

	Birth to 3 Mothers (n = 65)		Mothers with FAS/E (n = 30)	
	% or mean	(n)	% or mean	(n)
Race: African American/Black	48	(31/65)	3	(1/30)
White	29	(19/65)	53	(16/30)
Native American	15	(10/65)	37	(11/30)
Other (Hispanic, Asian)	8	(5/65)	7	(2/30)
Mean age at interview (years)	27.4	(65/65)	28.0	(30/30)
Has high school diploma	48	(31/65)	57	(17/30)
Not legally married at interview	97	(65/65)	77	(23/30)
Mean number of children	3.0	(65/65)	1.8	(30/30)
Mean age at first pregnancy (years)	19.7	(60/65)	18.0	(30/30)
Has children not living at home	55	(36/65)	54	(15/28)
Mean IQ	83.3	(47/65)	83.0	(28/30)
Was employed at interview	0	(0/65)	17	(5/29)
Was receiving public assistance at interview	83	(54/65)	82	(24/29)
Has driver's license	8	(5/65)	33	(10/30)
Personal History				
Has lived with alcohol/drug abuser	92	(60/65)	97	(29/30)
Has history of domestic violence	78	(47/60)	68	(19/28)
Was ever physically or sexually abused (as a child or adult)	92	(55/60)	77	(23/30)
Ran away as a child	59	(30/51)	63	(19/30)
Dropped out of school	75	(38/51)	67	(20/30)
Trouble With The Law				
Was ever arrested	95	(57/60)	50	(15/30)
Alcohol/Drug Problems				
Has history of alcohol abuse	65	(39/60)	70	(21/30)
Mean age first alcohol use (years)	15.7	(58/60)	15.5	(20/30)
Drank during pregnancy	79	(51/65)	40	(12/30)
Has history of drug abuse	100	(65/65)	70	(21/30)
Has history of prior alcohol/drug treatment	53	(32/60)	47	(14/30)
Birth Control				
History of problems using birth control	97	(58/60)	70	(19/27)

ences as their clients, including poverty, domestic violence, single parenthood and/or alcohol or drug problems themselves or within their families. Advocates in recovery have been so for over 10 years. The advocates receive extensive training, weekly individual clinical supervision, and participate in weekly strategy meetings.

For the research component of the project, mothers were recruited postpartum at the hospital of delivery using a one-page alcohol/drug screening questionnaire administered by a research assistant who was not part of the hospital staff (Streissguth, Grant et al., 1991). As Birth to 3 became known in the community, client referrals of alcohol or drug-abusing women who were not receiving prenatal care were accepted from professionals at health, social, and welfare agencies working with high-risk women. A total of 30 clients and 31 controls were enrolled at the hospital. Thirty-five clients were enrolled by community referral.

Although urine tests were not used for research screening, of the 65 mother/baby client pairs, 54 (83%) had had a urine screen for either the mother or the baby. Of these, 39 mother/baby pairs with at least one urine screen tested positive for illegal drugs (60%). Thus, the self-report screening and referral methods used by this study were more effective than were urine screens in detecting substance-abusing mothers. Furthermore, the procedures used here resulted in clients who had been willing to self-disclose their substance abuse in a confidential setting, and thus were more likely to be good treatment risks. The women enrolled in Birth to 3 had received few, if any, mental health services in the past and had not been evaluated for FAS or FAE.

The Intervention

The Birth to 3 model recognizes the importance of interpersonal relationships in women's addiction, treatment, and recovery. A woman's sense of connectedness to others is central to her growth, development, and definition of self (Miller, 1991; Surrey, 1991), and positive relationships, both with family members and within an intervention setting, are critical to successful drug abuse treatment for women (Amaro & Hardy-Fanta, 1995; Finkelstein, 1993). This interpersonal relationship aspect may determine whether or not a patient remains in an intervention (Barnard et al., 1988), and may be more critical to improvement than concrete services received (Pharis & Levin, 1991). Advocates in the Birth to 3 project provide a sounding board and the honest and consistent emotional support critical to women attempting to make fundamental changes in their lives.

The intervention model involved four basic steps: establishing the client-advocate relationship; identifying client goals; establishing linkages with service providers; and role modeling and teaching basic skills.

Advocates and clients began by getting to know each other immediately after the birth of the target baby, beginning to establish the trust that enabled them to work closely together for three years. This bonding process took months for those clients whose lifelong experiences of abuse and abandonment had taught them not to trust anyone. During this initial phase, the advocate addressed immediate problems such as obtaining clothes and diapers for the newborn, locating temporary housing, or assisting the woman in obtaining welfare benefits for the family. These activities demonstrated to the client very early in the project that the advocate cared and could be trusted to follow through.

The advocates worked within the context of the client's family, and established trust and rapport with the other children, the husband or significant other, and members of the extended family. As mothers, our clients are at the center of this network of relationships, in which everyone is involved in some way with their substance-abuse and related problems. They are all affected by changes the woman makes as she attempts to break long-established behavioral patterns.

Within one week after enrollment, the advocate met with her client to assess the family situation. The client identified her own most problematic issues using the "It Would Make a Difference Game," a card-sort needs assessment (Dunst, Trivette, & Deal, 1988; Grant, Ernst, McAuliff, & Streissguth, 1997). The client and advocate decided upon and recorded meaningful goals and the steps that could be taken to attain them, and together they evaluated and re-established goals and steps every four months. Using this concrete, dynamic and ongoing process, they developed plans realistic for both of them, in a way that gave the woman a voice and an opportunity to make her own decisions, and allowed her to observe and monitor her own progress.

Beginning at enrollment, the advocate contacted service providers with whom the client would be involved in order to establish a team approach to working with the client. The advocate conveyed clearly that her role was that of an individual case manager responsible for an individual client; helped the client articulate her objectives and commitment; and facilitated the development of a service plan. Service delivery systems with which advocates worked included child welfare, healthcare, drug and alcohol treatment, child development, mental health, educational, judicial and correctional systems. As confidentiality requirements at social service agencies limit the amount of information that can be shared, advocates asked clients to sign release of information forms when necessary.

The advocate acted as a liaison for communication within this working group in order to alleviate duplication of professional services, working at cross-purposes, or manipulation by the client. Clinic and agency effectiveness was improved when advocates managed the myriad complications (e.g., lack of housing, transportation) that would otherwise hinder or defeat a service provider's purpose. For example, drug and alcohol treatment in our state is a complicated process involving state-mandated assessments and paperwork. Advocates were very involved in helping clients negotiate these steps, and provided extensive practical assistance and emotional support to clients in a manner that could not be duplicated by service providers with high caseloads, specific agendas, and time constraints.

In appropriate situations, a "strong arm" in the form of a written contract proved to be beneficial for the client, the advocate, and the service provider. Advocates worked with clients and providers (e.g., landlords, judges, outpatient treatment counselors) to draw up agreements that defined explicit responsibilities and timelines. Clients were more likely to adhere to goals when they participated in establishing concrete, logical steps. The advocate could refer to the contract both in supporting her client and upholding the position of an agency. Personalized agreements heighten service providers' awareness of the possibilities of working successfully with this population.

The close proximity of the advocates to their clients' lives means that they are in a unique position to identify grave parenting problems in high-risk families that otherwise would have escaped detection from health and social service providers. Although one goal of the intervention is to promote a healthy relationship between the mother and baby and keep the dyad together, advocates do instigate removal of children from the home when necessary.

Role-modeling and teaching basic life skills were critical advocate strategies. It was clear that the clients' bleak backgrounds had done little to prepare them for adult life or parenting. For example, some problems with landlords and bill collectors were due to the fact that these women had never lived in a household that was "managed," nor had they had adequate training to prepare them for basic functioning within an economic system. Many of the women in the project had mothers who were alcoholic and/or drug abusers, and may themselves have experienced the effects of prenatal exposure to alcohol and drugs. In addition, cognitive impairment may have occurred as a result of their own years of substance abuse. Advocates found that the most effective teaching techniques with clients were those that were very explicit and concrete.

Advocacy is not a desk job, and advocates made frequent home visits, as determined by issues the client was working on. They provided transportation and found that time spent in the car with a woman was valuable because they could talk together at length with relatively little distraction.

Three general principles characterized the advocate/client relationship.

• Advocates worked with the understanding that relapse was to be expected among clients with a long history of drug or alcohol abuse; any difficult undertaking requiring a woman to make pivotal changes in long-established patterns of behavior may entail setbacks.

• Women were never asked to leave the project because of noncompliance, poor performance or relapse. This policy resulted in clients' increased ability to overcome embarrassment and humiliation after relapse and resume treatment more quickly and with greater determination. With the help of drug and alcohol treatment counselors, advocates used the experience of relapse to help clients examine events that triggered the setbacks and develop coping strategies.

• Conceptually, the intervention allowed for a gradual transition to occur from initial dependence on the advocate's assistance and emotional support, to a more independent, healthier lifestyle. This weaning process occurred as women became drug-free, began to trust in themselves as worthwhile and capable people, and learned the skills necessary to manage their lives. Success also depended on recognizing that not all such mothers would be capable of fully independent functioning; not all would be able to manage full custody of the target infant and all their children.

Intervention Outcomes

At the time Birth to 3 clients joined the project, their lives were characterized not only by substance abuse, but by the kinds of adverse circumstances that result from a dysfunctional upbringing and chaotic lifestyle. Table 1 presents the background characteristics of the Birth to 3 mothers.

After three years of advocacy services, we found the Birth to 3 approach to be effective in helping women enter alcohol/drug treatment, remain abstinent from alcohol and drugs, use birth control regularly, and become more involved with health and social services for themselves and their children.

Eighty percent of clients received some form of alcohol/drug treatment service over the 3-year project period, compared to 65% of controls. Fourteen clients (23%) entered and completed inpatient or outpatient treatment for the first time in their lives during the three-year intervention period. In contrast, none of the controls who went into inpatient or outpatient treatment during the same period were entering treatment for the first time. At the 36-month follow-up, 40% of clients were abstinent and had been clean and sober for at least six months compared to 28% of control mothers. Clients' self-reported use of birth control on a regular basis increased from 3% at enrollment to 73% after three years of advocacy services, while the control group increased from 12% to 52%. Clients were more likely than were controls (43% to 32%) to be using permanent (tubal ligation) or low maintenance (Norplant, IUD, Depo-Provera) birth control methods.

When clients who had spent more time with their advocates over the three years were compared with clients who were less involved, findings supported the conclusion that those who were more involved in the relationship aspect of the intervention were more likely to enter treatment, stay in recovery, deliver fewer subsequent drug-exposed children, and retain custody of the target child.

In summary, traditional drug treatment programs, therapy groups, or clinics simply are not equipped to manage the multiple and complex problems with which this high-risk clientele presents, nor do clients themselves have the resources, or skills to untangle and resolve these problems. The total cost of providing this advocacy in the Seattle area has been approximately $3,800 per year per client. This total cost is less than the cost of two days in intensive care should the mother deliver another alcohol or drug affected baby. Birth to 3 is an economical, practical model using paraprofessional advocates who can connect clients with necessary services while offering the critical element of ongoing personal support to clients and their families.

Applying the Birth to 3 Model to Mothers with FAS/FAE

The behaviors typically seen in adults with FAS or FAE mirror the types of behaviors advocates observed among many of their Birth to

3 clients. These include poor social and organizational skills, impulsivity, inability to understand logical consequences, inability to plan ahead, inadequate emotional control, poor judgment, and difficulty in recognizing and setting boundaries.

Treating adults impaired by FAS or FAE is not a straightforward process, and there has been little information written about it (Novick & Streissguth, 1996). However, strategies that have been proposed for working with an FAS/FAE clientele reflect the types of approaches that have been successfully implemented in the advocacy model.

For example, in the treatment setting, FAS/FAE patients seem to respond well to a mentoring, one-to-one relationship where they feel a personal bond with a staff member who acts as an advocate. The therapist/advocate can help the patient develop concrete, consistent rules that guide behavior in specific situations, instead of relying on the patient's ability to generalize what she learns and modify her behavior. Individualized one-to-one relationships allow opportunities for the therapist/mentor to role-play to develop a variety of typical scenarios, and to work out ways for the patient to respond appropriately.

In addition, clinicians working with FAS/FAE patients emphasize the importance of involving the family to ensure that there is understanding and support in the home environment. They have found that these patients are often unable to follow through on obtaining services on their own. Without a supportive and highly involved family member they will need intensive case management to coordinate the many services they need and should utilize.

We suggest that the Birth to 3 Model — a strategy for preventing FAS and FAE that has been shown to be effective in working with high-risk mothers — can be implemented with parenting women who themselves are diagnosed with FAS/FAE. The Birth to 3 Advocacy Model can link the highest risk mothers with the family planning and alcohol and drug treatment programs that are essential components of FAS prevention.

An advocate working in collaboration with a client, her family, and her network of service providers over a period of three years reasonably can be expected to accomplish the following intervention and prevention steps:

1. Obtain clinical evaluations for the diagnosis of FAS/FAE among clients and their children. Help affected families follow up on referrals made through the diagnostic clinic, and make linkages with appropriate community service providers. Assist with navigating paperwork and transportation to appoint-

ments. (See chapter by Clarren and Astley for a description of a model diagnostic program and how it works as an intervention and prevention tool.)

2. Help clients evaluate their family planning needs and assist in obtaining reliable, long-term birth control methods as appropriate. As role models and teachers, advocates convey to clients that they have control over their own reproductive capability. They are able to have an impact on clients' use of long-term birth control methods that require an understanding of the method, a careful decision, and follow-up on appointments.

3. Obtain DDD (Division of Developmental Disabilities) status as appropriate in order to secure a measure of financial stability for clients and their families.

4. If a client is abusing alcohol or drugs, assist in obtaining assessment for inpatient or outpatient treatment (including financial arrangements for treatment services). As appropriate, locate treatment centers where a client can enter with her children. Locate an appropriate aftercare facility and/or transitional drug-free housing. If a client is not able to attend treatment with her children, arrangements may have to be made for childcare.

5. Help to build or obtain a protective environment for clients and their children. This can include obtaining safe, stable housing for clients (ideally in supervised settings); teaching and role modeling of basic issues such as bill paying, food shopping, and hygiene; and overseeing home situations to assure safety and stability for the children. Overseeing home situations may include helping clients make careful decisions about their abilities to adequately care for all of their children, mediation with Children's Protective Services (CPS) and the courts, and communicating with and supporting foster families to assure stable placement.

6. Help clients establish a solid network of community service providers who will continue to work with them after the advocate's services are no longer available. Educate this network of providers. Professionals who are informed about FAS/FAE and the primary and secondary disabilities associated with these diagnoses provide support and guidance to their affected clientele and to the public.

7. Help to locate long-term mentors for clients. Family members or friends who have become exhausted or burned out in dealing with an FAS/FAE client may be willing to resume a supportive mentoring role after an advocate has helped a client make progress on the steps described above. The advocate can collaborate with this supportive person in identifying strategies that work well with the client.

FAS and the Social Security Disability Process: Navigating the System

Peter H. D. McKee

Introduction

For some people with Fetal Alcohol Syndrome, there may come a time when they consider applying to the Social Security Administration for disability benefits. The decision to apply or not, and the impacts of that decision on a person with FAS, their loved ones and medical providers, can have long-ranging positive and negative effects. The decision to apply for Social Security disability benefits involves many legal, social, medical, vocational and psychological considerations. Once a decision to apply for such benefits is made, the claimant faces seemingly insurmountable barriers of bureaucracy, delay, and medical and legal processing, which can defeat an otherwise entitled claimant. With the belief that knowledge is power, the following chapter is written for those with FAS, as well as their friends, relatives, counselors, and other health care providers. Armed with an understanding of the standards of disability to be applied to any claim for benefits, as well as an understanding of the bureaucratic process that must be negotiated, it is my hope that those involved, either directly or indirectly, in the process of applying for and assessing disabilities will be better able to insure that the Social Security Administration makes a fair and informed assessment of *all* information relevant to the claimant's impairments.

Two cautionary points: first, simply applying for disability benefits with the Social Security Administration does *not* entitle a person to those benefits. As will be described below, a very rigid and restrictive definition of "disability" is applied by the Social Security Administration. A claimant's financial need, the untherapeutic nature of the evaluative process, the "social/political" wisdom of Social Security's disability system play *no* role in determining whether or not a claim for benefits has met the legal standards of disability. Second, although claimants must show that their disabilities render them unable to perform any kind of work for a continuous period of twelve months, a finding of disability by the Social

Security Administration should not be seen by those with FAS or any other disability as forever branding these people unable to work for the rest of their lives.

Under current regulations, the Social Security Administration reviews each case every three years. Nobody applying for these benefits is served by defining their existence or their view of themselves by the opinions reached by the Social Security Administration, whether benefits are awarded or not. In most cases, claimants applying for disability benefits are best served by living their lives, pursuing their treatment and sticking to their goals, independent of the outcome of any claim for disability benefits. In my eighteen years as a lawyer representing claimants before the Social Security Administration, I can not think of any client whom I helped to obtain his or her disability benefits who felt, by our joint efforts, that his or her goals in life finally had been achieved. As I frequently tell my clients, Social Security disability benefits are rarely a goal in themselves, but benefits can be a critically important tool that can serve a client well while he/she works with friends, family and health care providers in an ongoing struggle with his/her disability. The income provided by the Social Security Administration through its disability programs is never as much as one might make if one could work full-time, and the medical care provided usually does not cover all of the claimant's medical needs. However, through the assistance of Social Security's financial support and the medical coverage, many claimants are given vitally important support which allows them to strive to improve their own disabilities. Without this support, such continuing struggles might be beyond their means.

Basic Facts of the Social Security Disability System

The Social Security Administration, a federal agency under the umbrella of the Department of Health and Human Services, administers two disability programs. When people apply for "disability benefits" with the Social Security Administration, they may be encouraged to apply for benefits under both programs. Realizing the differences and similarities of these two programs is essential to a thorough understanding of how this "system" works, and of what benefits the applicant may be entitled to receive.

Title II Disability Insurance Benefits

The first disability program administered by the Social Security Administration is called "Social Security Disability Insurance

Benefits" (also known as SSDI, Title II, "Disability" or even "SSA"). This program, which I will refer to as "Title II," is, as its formal title implies, a disability insurance benefit. Like an insurance policy, claimants have to show that they are both "disabled" *and* have "paid their premiums" and gained their insurance coverage. The way "premiums" are paid is by the individual having a work history and paying Federal Insurance Contributions Act (FICA) taxes. Claimants must show that, from the date they first became disabled, they have paid into the Social Security system by working and earning approximately $500 per quarter in five out of the last ten years (twenty out of the last forty "work quarters"). Thus, what date a claimant asserts he or she became disabled is a critical determination which may have an important impact on whether the client is found eligible for Title II benefits, regardless of whether the client is now disabled. Title II disability benefits based on a parent's work history can also be awarded to people who have no work histories themselves but who have been continuously disabled prior to reaching age 22. For such people to receive Title II benefits, they must show that one of their parents had a work history, paid into the Social Security system and is either aged, blind, disabled, retired, or deceased.

Another feature of Social Security Title II disability benefits is that income and resources are not directly relevant to a claimant's eligibility for benefits. This is not to say that a person who is gainfully working can expect to receive Social Security disability benefits. However, if a person has an inheritance or investment income, not directly related to working, it should have no effect on the individual's eligibility for Social Security disability benefits.

If an applicant is found eligible for Title II disability benefits, that individual also will be eligible to receive Medicare insurance. However, Medicare insurance is payable only after two years from the date the claimant is found eligible to receive Title II monthly benefits. In addition, monthly premiums of approximately $43.80 currently are taken out of the claimant's Title II monthly disability check to pay for the Medicare coverage. Medicare does not pay for most outpatient medications.

The amount of monthly benefits payable to the claimant is based on the level of past earnings, the frequency of those earnings, and how recently those earnings were received. Without consulting Social Security's computer record of earnings, it is virtually impossible to tell what monthly benefit level an applicant might receive. In addition, retroactive benefits can be awarded up to one year prior to the date of application, if the claimant can show that he or she was disabled at that time. With the long delays with the application process, it is not uncommon to have a substantial back award in a given case.

Supplemental Security Income

The second disability program administered by the Social Security Administration is called "Supplemental Security Income Benefits." This program is also known as "Title XVI," Supplemental Security Income or "SSI." It is important to distinguish this program from the Social Security Disability Insurance Benefit Title II program. SSI is not like an insurance policy. Indeed, while claimants for SSI have to prove their disability by the same standard used in the Title II program, SSI applicants also must prove that they are "poor." SSI is similar to the public assistance disability program, in which the claimant must not have significant non-exempt resources or income. As a rule of thumb, a claimant for SSI may not have more $2,000 in non-exempt resources as an individual, or $3,000 in non-exempt resources as a married couple.

The original concept of the SSI program was to "supplement" the income of those disabled Title II recipients whose earnings records and resulting disability benefit payments were low. In the State of Washington, the current maximum benefit level paid on SSI alone is $512. Throughout the United States, the various states can voluntarily choose to supplement the SSI benefit level. Some states contribute several hundred dollars in matching funds to those provided by the Federal government. In those states, such as California, the benefit level on SSI is higher than is the level in those states that do not contribute.

With the receipt of SSI disability benefits comes a medical coverage — Medicaid. If an individual receives even a dollar of SSI benefits, that eligibility for one dollar of SSI benefits entitles a recipient to coverage by the Medicaid program.

Unlike the Social Security Disability Title II program, retroactive benefits can be paid only to the date the claimant first applies for SSI benefits. Retroactive benefits prior to the date of application on an SSI claim are not available.

Definition of Disability

At the heart of both Title II and Title XVI disability programs is the unique definition of "disability." Social Security's concept of disability is difficult to comprehend until one realizes that, although they use a word that is found in the English language and is pronounced like the English word "disability," Social Security's use of the term "disability" can best be understood as a unique foreign language. Only when claimants, their family and friends, and their health care providers understand Social Security's definition of "disability" can they seek to provide relevant information that will be essential to documenting a claimant's limitations.

Social Security's defines "disability" as follows:

> . . . the inability to engage in any substantial gainful activity by reason of any medically determinable physical or mental impairment which can be expected to result in death or which has lasted or can be expected to last a continuous period of no less than twelve months.

This definition of disability is not necessarily the same one used by state welfare disability programs, private disability insurance programs, the Americans with Disabilities Act, or other programs. It is its own definition, unique to the Social Security Administration, and it is the only definition applicable in a claim for disability benefits with this agency. The determination of whether or not a person is disabled under this definition is a legal determination. It is based on many factors, including medical evidence, age, education, and vocational factors. The fact that the claimant has been found disabled for another program, such as Labor and Industries, or a private insurance policy, does not prove that the claimant is "disabled" as defined by the Social Security Administration.

Put simply, and in possibly a slightly overstated fashion, the "disability" definition requires that a claimant applying for disability benefits must show that his or her physical and/or psychological impairments produce symptoms (which are reasonably related to their documented diagnosis) that preclude the individual from doing any job that exists in significant numbers in the national economy. It does not matter whether or not the claimant applying for disability benefits has ever done this work before. Also irrelevant are whether or not the claimant would like to do this work, whether or not the job would pay the claimant sufficient funds on which to live, or whether or not the claimant actually would get hired in today's job market. Simply put, it must be the medical problems and their adequately documented symptoms which preclude the claimant from doing all jobs.

However, it should be remembered that "substantial gainful activity" is based on a concept of full-time work. The fact that a person can work at a part-time job does not, in itself, preclude a finding of disability. Thus, consideration must be given to whether or not a claimant would be able to do full-time work, averaging between six and eight hours a day, five days a week. Threshold questions of stamina, reliability, and ability to handle the reasonable expectations and demands of any employer always should be considered.

Because the determination of disability is a complex legal decision, to be made by the Social Security Administration, a brief declaration by a health care provider that the claimant is "totally disabled" is neither a competent legal nor medical opinion. That same conclusion thoroughly documented by the medical findings and assessment of symptoms, however, could go a long way toward proving such a conclusion. The clinical observations and professional medical assessments can be clarified best by the claimant's medical providers.

A claimant also can be found eligible for disability benefits if he/she meets the criteria listed for specific medical conditions in the "Listing of Impairments" of the Code of Federal Regulations (CFR). In the Appendix to this chapter, I have attached the part of the CFR that lists the criteria for "Organic Mental Disorder," the listing most likely to be relevant to FAS. Most people who are found eligible for disability benefits do not meet these more restrictive criteria. If a claimant's medical condition and accompanying symptoms can be said to "meet or equal" a described "listed" impairment, regulations provide that such an individual will be found disabled regardless of their age, education and work experience. Because these criteria were based on the *Diagnostic and Statistical Manual of Mental Disorders, (Third Edition)* (DSM-III), the diagnostic tools currently being employed by the Social Security Administration are somewhat out of date. (There is now a fourth edition of DSM, known as DSM-IV.) However, as the criteria that are employed in assessing disability claims are based on DSM-III, it is important that the medical providers be able to provide information using the terminology of the DSM-III, rather than the more current DSM-IV.

The Application/Administrative Process

Initial Application and Reconsideration

The process employed by Social Security in evaluating a claim for disability benefits, whether it is a Title II or Title XVI claim, is the same. It can be best thought of as the process of climbing a ladder. Each rung up the ladder must be taken in order, with no rung being skipped. Jumping off the ladder after receiving a denial notice and starting over by reapplying will never get the claimant to the top of the ladder, where, by this analogy, benefits are awarded. Instead of reapplying, the applicant can climb to the next rung only by appealing the previous denial.

The first rung of the administrative process is called the Initial Application. All applications are made in writing, although frequently the application information is taken over the phone and a final "hard copy" is sent to the claimant for signature. In the numerous papers that must be completed in the initial application, the claimant must be bluntly and graphically honest about all the medical problems and must not be embarrassed to describe, in cold, hard details, all of the limitations his or her symptoms impose upon all aspects of a work setting, and in his or her daily life. The application for disability benefits is not a job interview, where it is common to minimize the negatives and glorify the positives. Only if all medical sources are identified, and all diagnoses and symptoms are bluntly and graphically described, can the claimant hope that the Social Security Administration will understand the limitations arising from the claimant's medical and/or psychological problems. The more detailed the information regarding the name, address and telephone number of medical providers, the greater will be the chances that Social Security Administration will locate these providers and obtain the necessary medical information which will prove the claimant's disability.

Once all of the paperwork is completed on the application, the actual papers are sent to a state agency called the "Disability Determination Service" (DDS). DDS gathers and assesses all medical information to determine whether or not the standards of disability have been met. Once a decision is made by DDS, a written "Initial Determination" will be issued. Usually captioned "Social Security Notice" or "Supplemental Social Security Income Notice," these written decisions will advise the claimant if benefits have been awarded. Assuming, for purposes of this article, that such notices deny the claim, the claimant has sixty days to exercise his/her right to climb to the next rung of the application ladder. Within sixty days, the claimant must request a "Reconsideration." This may be done by phone, but the claimant should assume the worst, and make sure that all such requests are done in writing and actually received by the Social Security Administration. It is a useful strategy for the claimant to photocopy and keep in an orderly fashion all papers given to the Social Security Administration.

At the Reconsideration level, a second look at the claim for disability benefits is made by a different person at DDS. If a claimant fails to make the "Request for Reconsideration" within sixty days of the date they received the Initial Determination, his or her claim will be denied for failure to pursue the claim in a timely fashion. *Always appeal an unfavorable decision well before the expiration of the sixty days.* If the claimant has seen new medical providers, or if additional medical records can be obtained to support the claim for benefits, those records should be described in the papers filled out by the claimant in a Request for Reconsideration. Claimants should also contact their medical providers to make sure that all records are provided which document their disabilities.

A written notice, similar to the first notice, but captioned "Notice of Reconsideration," ultimately will be sent, advising the claimant if his or her benefits have been approved or denied. Once again, to protest an unfavorable decision at this level, the claimant must file a protest within sixty days. At this next step, a written "Request for Hearing" should be filed within sixty days with the local Social Security office.

Administrative Hearing

If a claimant applying for disability benefits has been denied twice, the next stage of the appeals process will be an administrative hearing before a Social Security administrative law judge. While informal, and not similar to the popular images of trials in *Perry Mason* or *People's Court*, the administrative hearing can be quite intimidating. It is likely the first time that the claimant will be face-to-face with the individual making the decision in his or her case. Specific facts and information, relating to both the medical situation and the procedural history, may be centrally important, but this may not be understood by the claimant. It is common to find that the Social Security Administration has called medical and/or vocational experts who might testify and express opinions that contradict those of the claimant or even the claimant's treating physician. Vocational experts testify to hypothetical questions and might express their opinion that, despite the claimant's impairments, such an individual could reasonably be expected to do a variety of jobs.

The hearing gives claimants the best opportunity to present their own testimony and that of parents, spouses, friends and medical providers, to document both the diagnosis and the pervasive nature of the symptoms which are the basis of the claimant's disability. While the medical providers may be able to testify about their assessment as to diagnosis and the symptoms which lead to that diagnosis, non-medical "lay" witnesses, such as friends, relatives, or counselors, also can play critical roles. Such lay witnesses can act as the eyes and ears for the administrative law judge, to insure that the judge understands how the medically diagnosed conditions actually impact on the claimant's daily life. One way of understanding the role that lay witnesses can play is to think of such friends or relatives as video cameras, who have recorded the sights and sounds of the symptoms of the claimant's impairments. At the hearing, such witnesses can "play back," in graphic and bluntly honest detail, all of the limitations they have observed which, in any way, impact on the claimant's daily life and ability to work.

Specifically with respect to FAS, the wide range of the claimant's symptoms should be fully described by the witnesses at the hearing. The claimant's limitations in handling stress, maintaining stamina in work production or pace, the claimant's reactions to expectations of production, as well as limitations of concentration should be described, if relevant. The manifestations of cognitive impairment and confusion, memory problems, limitations of verbal communication, comprehension, limitations in response to stimulus, impulsivity, poor judgment, as well as any other symptoms which can be documented should be graphically and bluntly described.

The presentation of live medical testimony at the hearing from the claimant's doctors can be quite helpful, but is often difficult to arrange, if for no other reason than the doctors' busy schedule. From the very start of the filing of a claim for disability benefits, supportive health care providers should be encouraged to submit copies of all medical records, as well as a detailed narrative report summarizing their findings. Test results, counseling notes, school records, as well as other records which may have developed over the years, might well be compelling evidence to document the disability based on a diagnosis of FAS. Remember that it is the symptoms of a diagnosed condition, and not the mere diagnosis, that determine the severity of a person's limitations and any eligibility for disability benefits.

Decisions as to the strategy of presenting information at a hearing need to be made in advance. It is not uncommon for the claimant to excuse himself or herself while witnesses testify about the nature and severity of the claimant's impairments. Considerations need to be made as to the therapeutic impact of the blunt and graphic testimony from friends or relatives who focus solely on the negative limitations imposed by the claimant's impairments.

Legal Representation

Legal representation at the administrative hearing frequently is critical to insuring the presentation of the strongest possible case. While Social Security disability law is not one generally practiced by most lawyers, in most large cities there are experienced practitioners who regularly appear before the Social Security Administration at disability hearings. Most experienced practitioners take such cases on a "contingency basis." This means that the lawyer seeks no payment for his or her fee unless he or she is successful in gaining the claimant his or her benefits. Usually a lawyer's retainer agreement provides that the lawyer is to be paid 25% of the retroactive award that is paid in a successful case with the fee not to exceed $4,000. All attorney's fees to be charged must be approved in writing by the Social Security Administration, even if both the lawyer and the client agree to the fee. If a claimant seeking legal representation is unable to locate a lawyer in his or her area, the National Organization of Social Security Claimants' Representatives (NOSSCR), located at 6 Prospect Street, Midland Park, New Jersey 07432 (1-800-431-2804), has a free nationwide referral service.

Posthearing Appeals

In most cases, the administrative law judge will not announce his or her decision at the end of the hearing, but will take the case "under advisement" and issue a written decision several weeks after the hearing. If the decision is unfavorable, further appeals may be taken, within sixty days, to the last administrative level, called the Appeals Council. This final branch of the Social Security Administration is located in Falls Church, Virginia, and the review is done solely on the evidence presented at the administrative hearing, along with any written legal arguments that are submitted to the Appeals Council.

If the case is again rejected by the Appeals Council, the claimant has sixty days to file a formal appeal in federal district court. Most lawyers are hesitant to take on a new case for the first time after it has been denied by the Appeals Council because the lawyer has had no input into the preparation or presentation of the case to that point. Any federal court appeal will be limited to the records of the case up to that point.

Conclusion

The process of applying for Social Security disability benefits can be an overwhelming and prolonged effort that can appear insurmountable. Many of the symptoms of FAS make climbing this mountain far more difficult for those with FAS than it would be for the average, unimpaired person. The best opportunity to present a comprehensive claim for benefits can be achieved only through the team efforts of the claimant, family and friends, health care providers, and, at times, the claimant's legal representative. Because the Social Security Administration has no specific FAS criteria of disability, each claim necessarily will include efforts to educate the Social Security Administration and, if necessary, the administrative law judge, as to the nature of FAS in general, and, more importantly to, the specific manifestations of the symptoms in the given claim for benefits. With perseverance, determination, and attention to the details of the process, the seemingly insurmountable mountain called Social Security disability can be climbed.

Appendix 1

Code of Federal Regulations, Volume 20, Chapter III, Part 404, Subpart P (4-1-95 Edition)

12.01 Category of Impairments — Mental

12.02 *Organic Mental Disorders:* Psychological or behavioral abnormalities associated with a dysfunction of the brain. History and physical examination or laboratory tests demonstrate the presence of a specific organic factor judged to be etiologically related to the abnormal mental state and loss of previously acquired functional abilities.

The required level of severity for these disorders is met when the requirements in both A and B are satisfied.

    A. Demonstration of a loss of specific cognitive abilities or affective changes and the medically documented persistence of at least one of the following:

        1. Disorientation of time and place; or

        2. Memory impairment, either short-term (inability to learn new information), intermediate, or long-term (inability to remember information that was known sometime in the past); or

        3. Perceptual or thinking disturbances (e.g., hallucinations, delusions); or

        4. Change in personality; or

        5. Disturbance in mood; or

        6. Emotional lability (e.g., explosive temper outbursts, sudden crying, etc.) and impairment in impulse control; or

        7. Loss of measured intellectual ability of at least 15 IQ points from premorbid levels or overall impairment index clearly within the severely impaired range on neuropsychological testing, e.g., the Luria-Nebraska, Halstead-Reitan, etc.;

AND

    B. Resulting in at least two of the following:

        1. Marked restriction of activities of daily living; or

        2. Marked difficulties in maintaining social functioning; or

3. Deficiencies of concentration, persistence or pace resulting in frequent failure to complete tasks in a timely manner (in work settings or elsewhere); or

4. Repeated episodes of deterioration or decompensation in work or work-like settings which cause the individual to withdraw from that situation or to experience exacerbation of signs and symptoms (which may include deterioration of adaptive behaviors).

Representing the FAS Client in a Criminal Case

Jeanice Dagher-Margosian

Introduction

In February, 1995, I was asked to represent a 20-year-old man affected by Fetal Alcohol Syndrome (FAS) in a criminal appeal. The young man had been convicted by plea of criminal sexual conduct. His parents felt that the trial attorney did not understand the social and intellectual functioning of their son, whom they had adopted at birth. Consequently, the court originally had not been told about FAS, nor about how it affected their son's mental state.

In the state where the prosecution took place, there was no legal precedent which included FAS as a relevant factor. Thus, through the significant and interesting case described above, I became familiar with FAS as it impacts a criminal case. Through this experience, it became clear to me that Fetal Alcohol Syndrome is a significant factor in the crimes of many of those accused; it is a condition which affects a person's ability to plan conduct or, conversely, to resist impulse. As a direct or indirect consequence, many of these individuals find themselves in the criminal justice system at some point in their lives. Yet, a great many of those prosecuted either should not have been convicted, sentenced to traditional punishment, or both. Why is this? First, FAS may negate the "guilty mind" requirement essential to establishing legal culpability.[1,2] Second, it is not clear that incarceration is of any value in experientially punishing the FAS offender, or in assuring the community that he or she will not be a threat to public safety upon release.[3]

This chapter will look at some of the areas where FAS evidence might be pertinent in the preparation and presentation of a criminal defense. As the body of knowledge about FAS grows, so too must discussion among those concerned with the legal representation of individuals affected by it. It is imperative that legal professionals be cognizant of the unchangeable reality of the FAS client's singular circumstances as he or she is subjected to the criminal justice system.

Identification

FAS may be identified initially by the presence of some or all of a number of distinct physical characteristics. A number of these have been documented by researchers; a few are growth deficiency (height and weight), absent or nearly absent philtrum (groove above upper lip), thin upper lip, ear irregularities, and indistinct nose which is small and has a low bridge. They often are hyperactive and have poor attention spans. Individuals affected by FAS have small brain sizes, brain malformations, delayed development, and some level of mental retardation and learning disabilities (Streissguth, LaDue, & Randels, 1988).

As children grow into adults, their hyperactivity evolves into problems of distractibility, inability to attend to relevant information, and, conversely, the inability to ignore irrelevant information (LaDue, Streissguth, & Randels, 1992). Individuals with FAS also often have trouble with interpersonal relationships and daily living skills. They are unlikely to have successful social relationships; this is likely related, at least in part, to an inability to listen and respond appropriately to others, to a tendency to interrupt with unrelated comments, and to a tendency to talk a great deal without communicating any real thoughts or information.

Attorneys should look for the above physical, intellectual and behavioral characteristics. An attorney always should investigate the client's family history for maternal alcohol abuse during pregnancy. In addition, a poor school history, placement in special education, and an inability to complete tasks should bring up the possibility that FAS impacts the client's case. Clients of concern should be referred to a specially trained physician who can make an FAS diagnosis.

Relevance of FAS to Investigation, Trial, and Sentencing of the Affected Client Trial Phases

In general, trials have four major phases: investigation, pre-trial, actual trial (or plea), and sentencing (if there is a conviction). The question of a client's mental functioning is important at all of these stages. It may be relevant for appeal purposes as well. Some ways in which defense of alcohol-affected clients might be benefited by expert testimony or other information on Fetal Alcohol Syndrome are discussed below.

Confessions

A very early, powerful part of the state investigation of a criminal case is police questioning. Obviously, this often results in an incriminating statement by the suspect, which gives rise, in turn, to a criminal prosecution. Confessions are a very important part of the prosecution's arsenal; what could be more compelling than a defendant's own statement that he or she committed the charged acts? All too frequently, criminal defense attorneys do not become involved with a case until after the filing of criminal charges and cannot intervene in the questioning.[4] As a result, inculpatory statements may be made by suspects which later support arrest and prosecution. It is imperative that attorneys become involved in a case at the earliest possible time and scrutinize the circumstances under which any confessions are obtained.

Right to Remain Silent and Right to Counsel

In situations where an individual is approached by police for questioning, even when police stress that they do not suspect the individual, but only believe that he or she may have "important information" about a crime, the individual may remain silent and avoid self-incrimination.[5] *This is a fundamental constitutional right* which is available to a suspect from the very inception of a criminal investigation.[6, 7]

Individuals with FAS are vulnerable to manipulation and coercion by police in a far greater way than are those not affected. These clients frequently are impulsive and not socially inhibited. In addition, socialization is most often at children's age levels, even when individuals are actually much older. For example, in one study, individuals with FAS generally functioned at a level of 6 years, 7 months even though the median age was 16 years, 5 months (Streissguth, LaDue, & Randels, 1988).

The governing query in determining the constitutional validity of a confession is whether the acts were admitted to voluntarily *and understandingly.*[7] When the capacity to fully understand the consequences of making an incriminating statement to police is compromised or inadequate, the statement can be excluded from evidence.[8]

Methods of Questioning

Police questioning frequently is based on achieving a rapport with the suspect and making the individual think that police are not necessarily suspicious of him or her. Some examiners call this using "minimizing themes" or the "false friend" method. Police might ask in a criminal sexual conduct investigation, for example, "Have you ever fantasized about showing your penis to a girl, not that it is something you would do, but more like just a daydream?" It is easy to see that this is an effective technique for engaging a suspect in a conversation which will result in an inculpatory statement.

The common trait among individuals affected by FAS of trusting persons in authority and the desire to please others may easily result in self-incrimination. Disturbingly, the truth of a self-incriminating statement is questionable, due, in part, to the tendency of FAS clients to have stronger expressive language skills than receptive language skills. They may speak and sound better than they are actually able to comprehend. They may also have difficulty with short-term memory (Malbin, 1993). For this reason, attorneys should consider the fact that some clients can be led into making statements about supposedly past conduct that they literally cannot remember.

Another interrogation technique is isolating the suspect from family and friends. He or she may be kept in a small interrogation room for hours without contact with anyone other than police. With no witnesses and often with no recording of the interrogation, police question the suspect and attempt to obtain a confession. Promises that the individual will be free to leave, or that one or more charges or potential charges will be dropped once a statement is made are not uncommon. [9, 10]

Another tactic is to have a youthful individual's parent present when implied or express promises are made. The parent may place pressure on the suspect to talk to police, believing that if this is done, release will follow. Confessions may result from this method, although this tactic has been disapproved by the United States Supreme Court. [11]

Advice of Rights

Police must advise those being questioned of their constitutional rights prior to questioning. These are read from a card, and/or suspects are read the rights from a form which they are often asked to initial or sign.

It is obvious that many FAS individuals being questioned in a station house setting or in a police car, without a parent or other support person, may not be able to discern the meaning of their advice of rights, and, in many if not most instances, will not have the ability to waive them voluntarily. If a person later charged with a crime does not have the capability of understanding what these rights mean and that the rights may be asserted at any time, the advice itself is meaningless.

It is not the boilerplate recitation of a suspect's constitutional rights which satisfies the requirements of *Miranda v. Arizona.* [12] Rather, it is the individual's ultimate ability to avail himself or herself of those rights, if that is the suspect's choice, which is the basis for assessment of police compliance. Such understanding will not be present if an individual does not have the ability to appreciate the import of the rights given by police. Thus, it is important for an attorney, parent or guardian to accompany an FAS client into an interview. At a minimum, this insures that a witness is present to document police questioning techniques. Improperly obtained confessions can occur whether the interview is at the police station or somewhere else. The key is if questioning takes place in compulsive and "police-dominated atmosphere."[13]

Legal Responsibility and Competency

The law has long acknowledged that an individual must have both a criminal mind and commit a criminal act (mens rea and actus reus) before being found legally responsible for prohibited conduct. Accordingly, when defendants either do not understand what they do, or cannot control their actions, they are not guilty of a crime. Additionally, if a client is not able to understand the nature of the proceedings or to assist the defense attorney at the time the state proceeds against him or her, the defendant may be incompetent to stand trial.

Insanity, or lack of requisite mental capacity, must not be confused with competency, which is governed by different law. Insanity relates to the Defendant's mental state *at the time of the alleged criminal act*, i.e., if the Defendant (1) did not know the difference between right and wrong, or (2) did not know what he or she was doing at the time of the criminal act, or (3) even if the defendant did know these things but could not control himself of herself, the Defendant may assert a viable insanity defense. While insanity is an affirmative defense subject to a controlling statutory time frame, competency is a fundamental due process requirement.[14] It may be raised at *any* time during criminal proceedings.[15, 16] Further, competency is so critical to the very legitimacy of a proceeding that it is not solely the defendant's burden to raise or waive it (as exculpating evidence, affirmative defenses such as insanity, or objections would be). There can be no criminal proceedings against a defendant who is incompetent; it goes to the *rightfulness of any prosecution at all* rather than to the question of guilt or innocence.[17]

The diagnosis of FAS raises numerous questions about the fairness of the proceedings relative to legal responsibility and competency. How can a defendant form the requisite intent for the criminal offense if he or she does not appreciate the wrongfulness of the act due to learning and memory difficulties? Or, where an act requires a specific intent (a requirement in some crimes that the defendant not only intended to do the act, but also intended that the prohibited result occur), does an individual with FAS have that kind of forward thinking and planning ability? A defendant may not be capable of having the scienter or intent required to commit a punishable criminal act, especially if it requires a showing of specific intent. He or she also may be incompetent to stand trial. Although those who are mentally ill are often brought to a state of competency within a period of treatment, with developmentally disabled individuals this will not occur.

If a client appears incompetent or insane (not legally responsible for criminal actions) an attorney may seek an order for a psychiatric exam. Generally, this is conducted by a state psychiatrist. If the state examination does not confirm incompetency or insanity, the defense attorney may request an independent examination. Obviously, if a defendant is indigent, this exam is problematic. The court must order payment for an expert; the expert, however, does not have to be one of the defendant's choosing.[18] Expert testimony from a mental health professional experienced with FAS is essential; the earlier it is sought out, the better (see chapter by LaDue and Dunne).

Other important uses of the expert diagnosis and evaluation during trial include supporting a defendant's credibility through explanation of characteristics of clients with FAS (e.g., they may sound more socially mature than they are, or may exhibit inappropriate demeanor, each of which may alienate a jury if not explained). Another possibility is supporting justification of an FAS client's actions, or explaining involvement in a criminal enterprise.[19] Explaining the defendant's mental functioning to prosecutors may result in an advantageous plea bargain or sentence recommendation whereas the same may not have been possible without this information.

Sentencing

FAS can be argued as a factor to support mitigation in sentencing. Once an FAS diagnosis is confirmed, the defendant's culpability can be diminished significantly for purposes of punishment.[20] If a defendant is affected by FAS, this is extremely relevant to the question of whether incarceration is proportionate and productive.[21]

An eloquent example of a court's acknowledgment of FAS as a powerful sentencing factor is found in *Rose Abou*, supra. There, the trial judge, Judge C.C. Barnett, heard extensive evidence detailing the defendant's impairments as they related to her tendency to commit assaultive offenses. He observed that due to the defendant's prenatal brain damage from maternal alcohol abuse, frustration, followed by over-reaction through violence, was characteristic for her. No amount of traditional punishment through incarceration would alter this pattern. Rather, the court placed Ms. Abou on probation for three years and imposed a tightly structured rehabilitation program, including supervised living, education in basic life skills, and alcohol and drug treatment. In doing so, Judge Barnett refused to impose a term of incarceration as punishment, even though it was argued that this was necessary to deter others from similar conduct:

> It is, I believe, simply obscene to suggest that a court can properly warn other potential offenders by inflicting a form of punishment upon a handicapped person who has, indeed, committed an offense for which some sanction must follow. That is not justice. That is unthinking retribution. If it were inflicted upon Ida Abou she could not fully comprehend it or possibly learn from it. Id., 4.

These are thoughtful judicial actions which properly recognize the impact of FAS on an individual's ability to conform to societal norms, or to learn from traditional punishments. (see chapter by Barnett) However, such decisions are not yet common.[22] One reason for this situation is the widespread but incorrect belief among people within the criminal justice system that prisoners can receive "education" and "therapy" while incarcerated. Available information indicates, however, that these remedial avenues are not easily entered into within the prison system. Further, in many prisons, the only therapy for assaultive and sex offenders is group therapy. This type of cognitive "talk" therapy is not useful to clients affected by FAS. Due to the memory and learning problems of clients affected by FAS, little or no benefit can result from this approach. For this reason, experts in FAS diagnosis and treatment hold the view that prison is inappropriate for FAS offenders (Clarren & Streissguth, 1995). Further, it is likely that FAS offenders will learn additional deviant behaviors if placed in a prison setting. They learn experientially and the chances are high that they will be victimized. They are likely to repeat, upon release, the negative behaviors to which they were exposed in prison.

Conclusion

This chapter only begins discussion about Fetal Alcohol Syndrome and the many criminal defendants impacted by it that must take place in criminal tribunals. The presentation of FAS-based defense arguments is crucial to constitutionally acceptable outcomes for criminal defendants with FAS. Our criminal justice system is based on true adjudication and fair penalties, and it must be true and fair for all of us. Increased awareness of FAS by judges, prosecutors, and defense counsel is necessary so that affected individuals will no longer be subjected to the "unthinking retribution" that has been prevalent in the past.

Notes

1. It is axiomatic that there can be no crime without criminal intent, or scienter. "A criminal intent is a necessary ingredient of every crime." *Pond v The People*, 8 Mich 149, 174 (1860). See also, *Morrisette v. United States*, 342 US 246; 72 S Ct 240 (1952). (US Supreme Court reversed a conviction for knowingly stealing and converting property of the United States when the defendant had taken spent bomb casings that appeared to be abandoned; the defendant did not know the Government owned the casings, and thus did not meet the requirement for criminal liability, i.e., "an evil-meaning mind and an evil-doing hand.")

2. "Scienter is not a word of mystery, or magic meaning. It is merely an expressive word . . . signifying in the connection commonly used that the alleged crime or tort was done designedly, understandingly, knowingly, or with guilty knowledge." *People v. Gould*, 237 Mich 156, 164 (1927).

3. The Eighth Amendment guarantee against cruel and unusual punishment now governs the imposition and evaluation of all prison terms under both state and federal law. Sentences must be proportionate to both the offense and the offender. US Const, Am VIII; *Solem v. Helm*, 463 US 286; 103 S Ct 3001, 309; 77 L Ed 2d 637 (1983).

4. In Michigan, for example, appointed counsel often is not provided for defendants until after arrest and pre-trial arraignment at which the defendant is read the charges against him or her.

5. Investigators also may indicate that if an individual speaks with them, the individual will be "let go" or police will be helpful in any ensuing prosecution. Remaining silent is always a better course than is making a statement before consulting with defense counsel.

6. In the case referred to above, counsel was not retained until well after a statement was made by the defendant. In fact, he had willingly presented himself at the police station, accompanied by his father. His father, believing it was best to cooperate with police, allowed the defendant to speak with the investigator without a parent or other witness present.

7. US Const, Am V, XIV.

8. *Spano v. New York*, 360 US 315; 79 S Ct 1202; 3 L Ed 2d 694 (1966).

9. Baker, L. (1983). *Miranda: Crime, Law and Politics*, 13. New York: Atheneum.

10. *Culombe v. Connecticut*, 367 US 568; 81 S Ct 1860, 1862-1863; 6 L Ed 2d 1037 (1961). Where suspect had mental age of nine, was suggestible and easily intimidated, and questioned largely in isolation while in custody, the

Court reversed his conviction, noting that "what actually happens behind the closed door of the interrogation room is difficult if not impossible to ascertain . . . The prisoner . . . knows that no friendly or disinterested witness is present — and the knowledge may itself induce fear."

11. Id. (The suspect's wife was present and placed pressure on the suspect to confess; this was held to be one of the factors which rendered "the proceeding an effective instrument for extorting an unwilling admission of guilt," which violated due process protections.)

12. 384 US 436; 86 S Ct 1602, 16 L Ed 2d 694 (1966).

13. *Illinois v. Perkins*, 496 US 292; 110 S Ct 2394, 2397; 110 L Ed 2d 243 (1990). Warnings must be given when a person is either in custody or otherwise feels deprived of freedom of action in any significant way. See *Berkemer v. McCarty*, 468 US 420; 104 S·Ct 3138; 82 L Ed 2d 317 (1984).

14. US Const Am V, VI XIV; Const 1963, art 1, 17.

15. Drope v. Missouri, 420 US 162; 95 S Ct 896; 43 L Ed 2d 103, 113 (1975).

16. Riggins v. Nevada, US; 112 S Ct 1810; 118 L Ed 2d 479 (1992).

17. In Godinez v. Moran, US, 113 S Ct 2680; 125 L Ed 2d 321 (1993), the United States Supreme Court made clear that when a criminal defendant waives his or her rights, that defendant must be competent at the time of the waiver. This includes such trial-level strategic decisions as what defense to put on, and how, " . . . and whether to raise one or more affirmative defenses."

18. In *Ake v. Oklahoma*, 470 US 68; 105 S Ct 1087; 84 L Ed 2d 53, 61 (1985), the US Supreme Court held that in an insanity proceeding, where the mental state of the criminal defendant was a significant factor in his defense, failure to provide him with a court-appointed expert was a due-process violation. Much emphasis in the opinion is placed on the defense having the proper tools to work with during a criminal trial.

19. An example is found in drug cases, where individuals with diminished mental functioning often are intimidated or bribed by dealers to participate in drug sales. A related defense tactic would be to bring in FAS evidence to support an entrapment theory, meaning that the defendant was entrapped by the state to be involved in one or more drug transactions.

20. Expert testimony generally may be ordered and received by the court at any phase of the proceeding, even if only used for sentencing purposes .

21. Regina v. Ida Rose Abou, LC No. 17459, 17460T, 1/24/95.

22. At least one court has considered FAS a reason to increase a sentence. In *US v. Janis*, 71 F 3d 308 (8th Cir. 1995), the victim was affected by FAS and considered by the court to be unusually vulnerable. The court used this as a reason to adjust the sentence upward by two levels of the sentencing guidelines.

A Judicial Perspective on FAS:
Memories of the Making of Nanook of the North

The Honourable Judge C. Cunliffe Barnett

Geoffrey was nine when I first heard about FAS from Dr. David F. Smith at a workshop at 100 Mile House, a small community in South Central British Columbia.

A few months later, in October 1981, I was the presiding judge during a child protection hearing at 100 Mile House. The Superintendent of Child Welfare had apprehended Geoffrey from his alcoholic parents and sought a wardship order. A parade of witnesses told me that Geoffrey was clearly a child with special needs, that many approaches and programs had been tried, and that nothing seemed to work. I suggested that Geoffrey be assessed by Dr. Smith; the social workers were reluctant but it did happen. Dr. Smith's report is dated January 29, 1982. It was written after he and his associates observed and examined Geoffrey during the course of a two-week stay at the Health Centre for Children in Vancouver. Dr. Smith said "Geoffrey clearly has the Fetal Alcohol Syndrome." He suggested Geoffrey had "minimal brain dysfunction" and said "he will never achieve average abilities," but was "trainable." I made a permanent wardship order in February 1982 and then took the extraordinary step of writing to the Superintendent of Child Welfare and sending him a transcript of my decision. I did not want Geoffrey's plight to be overlooked.

But it was.

I next saw Geoffrey in 1993. He appeared in court charged with a number of major sexual assaults upon young boys and a handicapped young woman. I learned then that Dr. Smith's recommendations had been ignored or overlooked, that Geoffrey mostly had been "cared for" during the previous 11 years in "different types of group homes," that he was functionally illiterate, and that he had "no insight into the seriousness of his offenses" and blamed his victims.

In June 1994, Geoffrey was detained in jail while awaiting trial. Being a small and needy man, Geoffrey was repeatedly sexually violated and victimized until he was released in February 1995.

Geoffrey's story is not a happy one, but it is absolutely true and, I fear, not unique or even unusual. *Fantastic Antone Succeeds* (Kleinfeld & Wescott, 1993), a wonderful book, tells of successes in the lives of young people afflicted with FAS. I have no such stories to tell. Echoes of Geoffrey's story permeate the pages that follow.

During the past fifteen years I have heard quite a number of cases in which persons afflicted with FAS/FAE played significant roles. These have included youths charged with crimes, men and women charged with crimes, child welfare hearings, child custody contests, and a girl with FAS who was raped. She was required to testify and tell her story.

In December 1995 I decided to do a cross-Canada Quicklaw search: to pull up every available decision with any mention of FAS or FAE. Some readers will find the results interesting — or perhaps, disconcerting:

> There were only 55 Canadian cases in which the decisions make some mention of FAS or FAE.

> Seventeen of these are criminal cases, 31 are child welfare or child custody cases, and seven of the cases mention FAS/FAE for incidental reasons only.

> There were 23 mentions in decisions from British Columbia, 11 mentions from the Yukon Territory, 6 mentions from Alberta, five mentions each from Saskatchewan and Manitoba, three mentions from Ontario, and one mention each from New Brunswick and Nova Scotia. There were no mentions from Quebec, Newfoundland, Prince Edwards Island, or the Northwest Territories.

> There were no mentions in the Supreme Court of Canada and only five mentions in all the Canadian Courts of Appeal (and two of those mentions are incidental/inconsequential).

A Canadian forensic psychiatrist has estimated that 30% of our prison population may have FAS/FAE. It is safe to say that judges encounter such persons frequently, recognize them seldom, and find that discouragingly few resources are available in any event.

Ida's case brought all of these unhappy truths together for me in January, 1995. My decision in that case is reproduced here. The decision was not written in obscure legalese; it can, I think, be appreciated by the average reader. I have edited the decision only very slightly for these pages. (Editor's note: We have edited this decision slightly as well.)

Text of the Decision

The stories heard by judges are endlessly sad and disturbing. Ida's story, which I shall recount on these pages, is one of the saddest and most disturbing that I have heard during more than 20 years of judging.

Ida is a small and artless woman, not quite 24 years old. She is a Sekani Indian whose home community is the Indian reserve at Fort Ware, British Columbia.

Life is harsh in Fort Ware, and Ida's life has been marked by an uncommon number of tragedies. Her father was killed in 1975. Her sister was sent to prison for manslaughter in 1992. Later in 1992 her sister was killed by the man who had killed their father. Other members of Ida's immediate family have been sentenced for violent offenses. All of the killings and other violent incidents were fueled by alcohol.

Ida was raised by her alcoholic grandparents.

Ida claims to have a Grade 2 education (or perhaps it was Grade 4 or 5 — she really cannot remember). She is mentally handicapped. Ida's school in Fort Ware was run by the Division of Indian Affairs until June 1994. The educational standards were notoriously and abysmally low. Services for students with special needs were essentially nonexistent.

Ida has given birth to seven children — it appears that all have FAS or FAE and all are "in care."

Ida's children demonstrate the fact that she is a severe abuser of alcohol. When Ida is under the influence of alcohol she has a distinct inclination to act impulsively and violently.

The author of a pre-sentence report written in August 1993 summarized matters by saying that Ida's life has been "punctuated with poverty, alcoholism, violence, and death." When that report was being prepared, responsible persons in Fort Ware expressed the thought that "it is as though she has never been taught right from wrong."

There is more.

Ida herself almost certainly is afflicted with FAS, a fact which apparently went unrecognized until a court-ordered report was written by Dr. Kerr in July 1993.

FAS has been the subject of comment in only a few reported Canadian court decisions (Joe v. Yukon Territory (1986) 5 BCLR (2d) 267 and R v. RBM (1990) 54 CCC (3d) 132). FAS is not well understood by most judges, lawyers, probation officers, corrections officers, social workers or other persons likely to encounter it in the context of the justice system.

It is not a new notion that the taking of strong drink by pregnant women endangers unborn babies. People understood this truth in biblical times, but ancient wisdom was largely forgotten or ignored until about 20 years ago, when the first reports of modern studies were published. We have now come to understand that fetal exposure to alcohol is the leading cause of mental retardation in Canada. Moreover, fetal exposure to alcohol causes actual brain damage and the long-term effects are more severe than are those of other drugs, including heroin and cocaine.

People whose brains were damaged by alcohol before they were born are entirely likely to have characteristics which will bring them into conflict with other persons and the criminal law or set them up to become victims of crimes, particularly sexual crimes. Ida is prone to becoming frustrated and then to over-react in impulsive, violent ways. Behavior like this is entirely consistent with her affliction and it is not merely willful misbehavior by a woman who refuses to mend her ways. Persons with FAS have brains which simply do not "work right." They cannot be made to learn and change by the punishments which are the traditional tools (or weapons) of our criminal justice system. They may however cope pretty well and be considered model inmates in the highly structured environments of prisons and penitentiaries.

Ida is in court today because I must sentence her for two criminal offenses:

1. Assaulting Myrna Charlie at Fort Ware on February 8,1994.

2. Assaulting and causing bodily harm to Robby Pierre at Fort Ware on February 12, 1994.

The circumstances of these offenses are not extraordinary. On February 8, 1994 Ida got into a trivial argument with another young woman, Myrna Charlie, who she then beat up. Ida put Myrna down and kicked her in the head. A few days later, at a time when she had reason to be upset with Robby Pierre who was making a drunken nuisance of himself, Ida grabbed a kitchen knife and slashed Pierre's leg with it. He was hurt, but not terribly seriously. Ida pled guilty to the assault upon Myrna Charlie. She was tried and found guilty of the assault upon Robby Pierre.

These offenses were not Ida's first. In September 1992 Ida got into a trivial argument with Christine Poole, who merely had wanted to borrow some cigarettes. When Christine departed the scene Ida grabbed a knife and followed her. Ida slashed Christine with the knife, and inflicted a significant wound. On that occasion Ida had been drinking home brew and was not sober. She was similarly under the influence when the present offenses were committed.

I sentenced Ida for the assault upon Christine Poole at Quesnel on September 28, 1993. The transcript of those proceedings was filed during the course of the present proceedings. It records the fact that in September 1993, officials within the Corrections Branch were unwilling to extend a helping hand to permit a form of sentencing that might have been constructive. I said that was "a shameful mistake" and predicted that the sentence I did impose would prove to be "inadequate." I was certainly right about that!

Mr. Justice David Vickers has recently spoken strongly about the difficulties FAS and other handicapped persons encounter in Canada. He says (in the case of Victor Williams) that our model of service delivery "is counter-productive, judgmental and non-supportive."

One real tragedy of cases like Victor William's, and Ida's, is that nobody made any effort to provide any meaningful help until it was, perhaps, too late. We must all pay a very real price for these and other similar failures, and persons whose handicaps might have been addressed are now stigmatized as criminals.

I do not mean to suggest that Ida should not be held responsible and sentenced for her actions. That is not the law in Canada and she clearly is capable of seriously threatening the safety and well-being of other persons. A judicial response is rightly demanded.

But what might be a fair, reasonable, and constructive response?

When crown counsel spoke to sentence before Justice Vickers in the case of Victor Williams, he said the court's principal consideration should be general deterrence. When crown counsel spoke to this case in Quesnel on November 30, 1994, I heard a similar submission. Justice Vickers rejected this concept in the Williams case, and rightly so. I reject it in the present case. It is, I believe, simply obscene to suggest that a court can properly warn other potential offenders by inflicting a form of punishment upon a handicapped person who has, indeed, committed an offense for which some sanction must follow. That is not justice. That is unthinking retribution. If it were inflicted upon Ida she could not fully comprehend it or possibly learn from it.

I believe that in sentencing Ida I must focus upon two essential needs:

1. It is necessary to provide a measure of protection for other persons.
2. It is necessary to provide a realistic framework for her possible "rehabilitation."

I remanded Ida into custody on November 3, 1994 after her trial at Fort Ware. I ordered that an updated and tightly focused presentence report be prepared. On a later occasion I wrote to the probation officer and counsel to request that a specific probation plan be incorporated in the report.

Mr. Kay put a lot of work into preparing his report. He makes sensible and constructive suggestions which I am pleased to be able to accept.

On November 30, 1994 I again remanded Ida's case — until January 24, 1995 in Williams Lake. There were two reasons for doing that:

1. I considered it essential that Ida complete a substance abuse treatment program and that the correctional center program mentioned in Mr. Kay's report was the most appropriate in her circumstances.

2. I hoped that during the remand period Ida could be seen and fully assessed by an FAS expert or experts. I mentioned the names of Dr. Christine Loock and Dr. Julianne Conry. I said I believed their recommendations would greatly assist any persons who might be tasked with supervising or assisting Ida during the term of a probation order.

I now have a report jointly authored by Christine Loock (a pediatrician and clinical assistant professor at University of British Columbia [UBC]) and Julianne Conry (an assistant professor in the Department of Educational Psychology and Special Education at UBC). This report contains a wealth of information. It is helpful to me and will, I very much hope, assist those who must help Ida and her children in the future.

Drs. Loock and Conry cannot be absolutely certain in their assessment of Ida. They observed a number of physical characteristics which strongly suggest FAS but these features, which may be very pronounced in childhood, are masked and subtle in adults such as Ida. They observed psychological indicators also but there are other possible causes of mental handicaps such as Ida's. Those other possible causes include events such as head injuries and there is a report that when Ida was a child she was hit on the head with a hammer by an abusive relative. Most importantly, Drs. Loock and Conry were not able to confirm the various reports that Ida's mother was actively drinking when she was pregnant with Ida. They say that "a definitive diagnosis cannot be made without prenatal history and documented maternal drinking." That is a very proper approach for conservative clinicians to take.

But while Drs. Loock and Conry cannot be definitive in stating the cause of Ida's handicaps, FAS is clearly the most likely cause and there is no doubt concerning the nature and extent of her handicaps. The observations of Drs. Loock and Conry are stark. Many of their recommendations are specific and practical. The recommendations, in their entirety, are

1. *Medical follow-up.* Follow-up is needed for the following concerns:
   a. Counseling with respect to family planning. Ida is at very high risk for very serious obstetrical complications if she were to become pregnant again, due to her large number of pregnancies in a short period of time. She is at high risk for having more children with FAS. She has apparently expressed the desire to not bear any more children. She would not be able to reliably use methods of birth control that depend on her ability to remember or plan ahead. Consultation with a gynecologist is needed to improve her general state of health.
   b. Ida's children, who are described as being alcohol affected, should be assessed and tracked, and have access to early intervention as appropriate.
2. *Cognitive limitations.* Ida has a significant mental handicap making her eligible for the benefits available to individuals with disabilities. She is severely limited in her understanding of what is being said to her or asked of her, with the result that her responses do not follow logically. She does not indicate (and maybe she is unaware) when she does not understand, but may respond affirmatively with "uh-huh." She has a severe memory deficit, such that basic requirements of day-to-day living must at times be very difficult. Basic academic skills are at the end of grade 1 level.

   Treatment and educational programs should be those designed for individuals with mental handicaps. These are characterized by concreteness, simplicity, constant repetition, and supervision.
3. *Alcohol and drug treatment.* Our understanding is that the program Ida is completing at the Burnaby Correctional Centre is only the first step in recovery for Ida. It is imperative that she not return to a drinking environment. (Mr. Kay's report indicates that the grandparents' home is the

center of a great deal of drinking.) She needs continued and intensive treatment. Due to her cognitive limitations, a Native culture/traditions approach may be most beneficial; her partner should attend with her.

4. *Care of her children.* Ida has a better chance of participating in the care of her children if her postpartum health improves and alcohol/drug treatment is successful. In the best of situations, special needs (FAS) children are very difficult to parent, but this is made all the more difficult when the mother lacks parenting skills. Ida says she would like a house and her children returned. It is unlikely that Ida could ever, independently, look after the needs of her children, but she should participate in their care. When queried, she said she did not find it difficult to care for children. By report, it does not appear she has ever had the responsibility of caring for her children. When the children have been in her grandparents' home, others have taken care of their basic needs. Attending a child care program, if designed for her ability level, would not be sufficient, but it would be desirable.

5. *Basic life skills.* The program described in Mr. Kay's report is appropriate (life-skills worker for four hours per day, five days a week), but there needs to be routine to fill the rest of the day. The life-skills worker can assist in putting such a routine in place. The life-skills worker is presumably skilled in teaching individuals with handicaps.

One important life skill is handling money. Living in Fort Ware has not provided Ida with basic learning and experience due to the fact that most purchases are made on a credit basis at the store. Ida does not have the basic computational skills to understand simple transactions. She does have a sense of greater and lesser values of things. For shopping, she could be taught to use a basic list (the same list every time) that will allow her to shop within a budget. Teaching Ida to use a calendar to schedule day-to-day tasks such as shopping and cleaning, and recreational activities, helps organize and fill her day.

The Association for People with Mental Handicaps could be helpful with regard to possible employment and recreational opportunities. Routine and repetitive jobs, such as cleaning, would be suitable. Ida says she likes cleaning. She learns best by being shown, rather than being lectured. Any job would require supervision and reminding, with an employer who understands Ida's limitations in language, memory, and basic literacy.

Ida does not seem to have a concept of "doing things for fun," but she expressed an interest in sewing and beading. She has taken an interest in Native culture through the Burnaby program and so programs at the Native Friendship Centre would support some of the gains made in Burnaby.

6. *Living arrangements.* The ideal living arrangement, sometimes provided for people with handicaps, would be an apartment complex where she is able to maintain her own suite, but where there is general supervision of the house. This would help control the problem of "friends" coming by late at night pressuring her to party. A curfew would be appropriate for the duration of her probation.

7. *Care of her grandparents.* Ida has a somewhat romanticized view of returning to Fort Ware which has been her home. Ida insists she needs to be back in Fort Ware in order to look after her grandparents who are "pretty old." She describes them as having physical problems (grandmother's problems with movement in hands and wrists, grandfather's problems in walking and moving about) and she worries that no one is helping them with their day-to-day needs: cutting firewood, washing, and cleaning. They do not know how to read and they can not use the washer/dryer. We understand that the band can provide some homemaker assistance, and so that situation is not as dire as she has convinced herself it is. As guardians of two of Ida's children, it would seem they are more capable than Ida believes. Also, she is unrealistic in her belief that the chief will have a house built for her, if she is there to ask for it; she needs to be told clearly that there is no way this will occur.

When Ida is residing in Prince George, regular day-only visits to Fort Ware (as there is no way to provide overnight supervision of drinking) could satisfy her concern and allow the Prince George program to be more successful.

8. *Need for regular assistance.* It is easy to anticipate that Ida could be set up for failure in meeting conditions imposed by the Court unless there is someone to help her meet those conditions — especially those conditions associated with remembering and reporting on a particular schedule. On a very frequent and repetitive basis, she needs to review what she is doing to meet the conditions and why these

conditions are imposed. Adults with the limitations of FAS often present as not appreciating the seriousness or the importance of conditions set out for them.

Clearly, prohibitions spelled out in Mr. Kay's report — especially abstaining from alcohol — are critical. As Ida seems to think that drinking in Fort Ware is less of a problem than drinking in Prince George, she may have a distorted idea that not all alcohol is equally harmful: beer, hard liquor, home brew, Lysol. With regard to all the prohibitions, they need to be spelled out in black and white. A simple message is best: e.g., If you keep drinking, you will die.

9. *Comprehending the meaning of violence.* Ida's apparent lack of remorse over the violent incidents, including expecting that her victim would forget about it, is something consistent with what is described for individuals with Fetal Alcohol Syndrome. In this instance, the additional factor is that violence has been a way of life for Ida. She describes how the Burnaby program has included anger management, but this is of minimal benefit when the violent episodes are associated with drinking. Obviously, the only hope in changing the cycle, is successful drug treatment."

The British Columbia Court of Appeal has said many times that persons who hurt other persons with knives or other weapons must anticipate serious jail sentences. Ida has been sentenced before for a violent offense. It would not be "wrong" if she were now sentenced to serve a year or more in jail. That, of course, would very obviously limit her freedoms for a period of time.

I do not intend to send Ida back to jail. Hers is a special case and counsel are agreed that it is appropriate today to suspend the passing of sentences and to place Ida on probation for three years. The terms of probation are very specifically intended to create a measure of structure in Ida's life. They limit her freedoms, but much less drastically than would jail sentences. There is some real reason to hope that the period of probation will be a constructive experience for Ida.

Part II of Ida's probation order, which might be called the short form of probation conditions, is reproduced below. The short form conditions are very deliberately stated in plain language and they are to be the conditions appearing in the probation order which Ida will sign.

I note that Ida's probation order does not presently contain alcohol counseling or curfew conditions. When she moves from the

Phoenix Transition House it may be appropriate to add such conditions to the probation order.

CONDITIONS OF PROBATION

1. You must report forthwith to a probation officer in Prince George.
2. You must report to your probation officer every day or faithfully meet with your AiMHi Life Skills Worker at least 5 days each week.
3. You must reside at a place in Prince George.
4. You will live at the Phoenix Transition House until Judge Barnett changes this order.
5. You must not drink alcohol. This includes whiskey, wine, beer, and home-brew.
6. You must never go to beer parlors, pubs or bars.
7. You must never carry a knife.
8. You must not go to Fort Ware unless it is necessary for you to appear in court there, or unless you go to Fort Ware in the morning and leave before it is dark that same day.
9. You must appear in court at Prince George on June 30, 1995 for a review of this order.

Conclusion

At this writing, 18 months have passed since I made the probation order in Ida's case. Things have not gone well. Ida pushed past the limits of those who tried to help her from the outset and within a very few months she was drinking, fighting, essentially homeless, and pregnant all over again. She gave birth to another afflicted child on November 12, 1995. She last reported to her probation officer in December 1995. She failed to attend a treatment center that she had promised and was required to attend in January 1996. She failed to attend court appearances and warrants have been issued for her arrest. Serious jail terms appear to be looming on Ida's horizon.

These developments in Ida's case have been discouraging. But one needs always to search for the silver lining and some other things happened following the decision in Ida's case.

The principal of the school in Fort Ware used the decision as a key element in his successful campaign to persuade DIA to fund the purchase of computers for the school. I am told that many children who were previously almost hopeless as students are now making truly remarkable progress.

I am told that my decision in Ida's case has been cited to judges in distant places and that it has helped them search and push for creative solutions.

The decisions in the cases of Victor Williams and Ida Abou received significant media attention in British Columbia and that was a real factor in persuading our judicial education committee that more judges needed to learn about FAS/FAE issues. In the spring of 1996 Dr. Diane Rothon made a seminar presentation to all the judges of the Provincial Court of British Columbia and she was exceptionally well received. To my knowledge, her presentation was a Canadian first.

Ida's children were all assessed. They are now all in permanent care and hopefully, their futures will be at least a little brighter.

When I wrote the decision in Ida's case I said that "one real tragedy of cases like those of Victor Williams and Ida Abou is that nobody made any effort to provide any meaningful help until it was, perhaps, too late."

On August 19, 1996, I received a probation officer's report concerning Alton who is the 19-year old son of a dedicated alcoholic and is also a sex offender. He has FAS "written all over him" but I am told that a formal assessment is being delayed because nobody seems to have the responsibility to get it done!

I am however a little encouraged by the case of Robert, age 16. He has incurred the wrath of quite a few judges and probation officers because he steals, will not obey probation orders, and appears very defiant, even in court. In late 1995 I was urged to "lock him up." I refused to do that and instead pulled out all the stops in an effort to get Robert admitted to a treatment center in Alberta. There was much pessimism, but Robert did go and it seems to have worked. I am told that a family associated with the treatment center has provided a home for Robert, that he is apparently happy, and that he is staying out of trouble!

In this work, the real success stories are hard to come by.

Legal Issues and FAS

Robin LaDue and Tom Dunne

Introduction

Fetal Alcohol Syndrome (FAS) and Fetal Alcohol Effects (FAE) are birth defects that result from prenatal alcohol exposure. As has been discussed in previous articles (Jones & Smith, 1973; Olson, Streissguth, Bookstein, Barr, & Sampson, 1994), FAS is associated with organic brain damage that has a negative impact on abstracting abilities, memory skills, information processing, comprehension of social rules and expectations, the ability to connect cause and effect, and the ability to learn from past experiences (LaDue, 1993; Olson, Streissguth, Bookstein, Barr, & Sampson, 1994; Streissguth, LaDue, & Randels, 1988). People with FAS often are described as being impulsive, having poor personal boundaries, and being easily influenced.

Many of these behavioral difficulties also are seen in people prenatally exposed to alcohol but lacking in the growth deficiency and facial dysmorphology necessary for a diagnosis of FAS. These people are often given a diagnosis of Fetal Alcohol Effects (FAE) (Clarren & Smith, 1978). In fact, patients with FAE, despite having, in general, higher IQ scores, commonly have more secondary disabilities and less access to support services than do patients with FAS. Given these factors, if appropriate interventions and structures are not put in place early in life and maintained across the life-span, many people with FAS/FAE are at high risk from birth through the adult years to become involved in the legal system.

In addition to the problems just discussed, people with FAS/FAE also tend to have a high need for interaction but lack the social or cognitive skills that help establish safe, long-term relationships. They may have difficulty distinguishing between strangers and "friends." They have difficulty structuring their own lives and behaviors. External, positive, consistent supervision and structure often is

Portions of this chapter have been reproduced and modified, with permission, from three articles (LaDue & Dunne, 1995; 1996-a; 1996-b) first published in the *FEN Pen* newsletter.

unavailable. Cumulatively, this set of circumstances leads to a not uncommon participation in petty crime, gang "involvement," most often as a "fringe" member or "gopher" and in a few cases, serious crimes. Once a person becomes involved in gang activity, the rate and severity of offending often increases. In some cases, unfortunately, the primary option for structure offered by society becomes that provided by penal institutions.

Fetal Alcohol Syndrome has had an odd place in criminal law. Once involved in the legal system, many people with FAS/FAE lack the ability to follow through on tasks in either a timely or reasonable fashion. Their ability to retain information is often compromised and they will commonly give whatever answer is "on the top of their head" or what they think is wanted. It is difficult for many professionals in the legal system to understand these problems and limitations as people with FAS/FAE often "sound" or "look" competent, capable, and rational. Their cognitive difficulties frequently are masked by their superficial verbal abilities. The actual abilities of people with FAS/FAE to truly understand the consequences of actions are frequently overestimated. Even more unrealistic expectations are often placed on people with FAE, given their sometimes normal IQ and lack of facial abnormalities or growth deficiency. The courts are not likely to recognize and understand FAE and, thus, are likely to impose detention/institution time rather than appropriate services.

Often, many affected people are not identified and diagnosed with FAS/FAE. Their cognitive difficulties and behavior problems are misunderstood and misinterpreted. They may be labeled stubborn, obnoxious, lazy, having antisocial personality disorder, or given other judgmental and not necessarily accurate labels. On the other hand, people who do receive the proper FAS/FAE diagnosis might have their possible psychiatric secondary disabilities overlooked or minimized. In this case, the false assumption is that *all* behavioral problems come from the neurological damage. Influencing and contributing factors such as early childhood neglect and abuse and individual personality differences may not be taken into account.

Legal Issues

Competency, capacity/diminished capacity, and decline/remand determinations are three of the most common reasons people with FAS/FAE are referred for psychological evaluations within the legal system. This chapter will discuss the particular issues raised when a person with FAS enters the legal system and faces these issues. The definitions of these legal terms presented in this paper are based on the Revised Code of Washington State. Definitions may vary from state to state and from state to federal statutes. However, the definitions in this chapter may be viewed as guidelines.

Capacity and Diminished Capacity

Arnie G. was a twelve-year-old African-American male who was referred for testing by his attorney, a public defender. Arnie had been picked up on several burglary charges and his attorney was concerned about his capacity to understand the reasons his behavior was considered wrong.

Arnie was the youngest of six children born to a woman who was reported to have used alcohol, cocaine, and other drugs during her pregnancy. Arnie's mother was unable to care for any of her children and they had all been placed into foster care. Arnie had run from his latest foster home several times and was, for the most part, living on the streets. He had not attended school on a regular basis for two years. He was described as having serious learning difficulties and had been in Special Education classes.

Arnie was given a complete psychological evaluation while he was in the juvenile detention center. His IQ scores were in the 60's and his achievement scores were below the first grade level. His adaptive behavior scores corresponded to average scores of five to six-year-olds. Arnie's verbal skills were poor and he was not able to articulate any understanding of why his behavior had been inappropriate.

Arnie was short, slight, microcephalic and had facial features consistent with Fetal Alcohol Syndrome (FAS). Because of his behavior, history of prenatal alcohol exposure, and physical attributes, Arnie was referred to a diagnostic clinic and subsequently was given a diagnosis of FAS.

Due to his low scores, poor verbal skills, and lack of abstracting abilities and understanding, it was found that Arnie did not have capacity to understand the charges against him or the legal process, and the charges against him were dropped. Arnie, however, did not fare well. He did not remain in the therapeutic foster home where he was placed, he continued to be involved in criminal activity, and, at age 16, finally was placed into long-term custodial care.

Michael J. was a single, white seventeen-year-old male when he was charged for the first time with a criminal offense: possession of stolen property. Concern was raised at the initial court hearing about Michael's reasoning ability. He gave a rambling explanation of how he had "not done anything wrong — the money was to be used to *help people." In addition, he stated how the "U.S. Government should declare war in order to save the rain forests."*

Michael's parents indicated he had recently been diagnosed with bipolar depression, although Michael disagreed with this diagnosis. Michael was given two independent psychiatric evaluations in preparation for Court, one by the defense and one by the prosecution. Both evaluators reached the same conclusion and diagnostic impression. Michael was found to be suffering from an Atypical Psychotic Disorder, which suggests severely impacted thought processes. It was determined that he had "diminished capacity;" he did not have the capacity to form the intent to commit a crime. The Court concurred and the charges against Michael were dismissed.

If it is found that a mental disorder causes sufficient problems in an individual such that they are unable to knowingly commit a crime, the individual is said to have "diminished capacity." Diminished capacity refers to a person's ability to establish either criminal intent or the motivation to engage in criminal behavior and to understand it as such. Diminished capacity is based on numerous factors such as the following:

- The defendant lacks the ability to form a specific intent due to a mental disorder not amounting to insanity;

- The cause of the inability to form a specific intent must be a mental disorder, not emotions like jealousy, fear, anger, and hatred;

- The inability to form a specific intent must occur at a time relevant to the offense;

- The mental disorder must substantially reduce the probability that the defendant formed the alleged intent; and

- The opinion from the evaluator must contain an explanation of how the mental disorder is responsible for the defendant's inability to form a specific intent; the explanation cannot simply be inferred.

A finding of diminished capacity requires the presence of a mental disorder. People who have a thought disorder, bipolar disorder, or other serious mental disorders may not have the full ability to recognize the concepts of right or wrong or be able to modify/control their behavior to meet community guidelines and expectations. They have diminished capacity.

Although the presence of a mental disorder is NOT part of the criteria for diagnosing FAS, secondary psychiatric disabilities frequently occur. Common psychiatric diagnoses associated with FAS include high-functioning autism, borderline personality disorder, depression, attention deficit hyperactivity disorder, and antisocial personality disorder. Periodic episodes of psychosis have been noted less frequently. With the exception of psychosis and autism, these diagnoses are unlikely to fit the criteria for diminished capacity. FAS itself is not recognized as a mental disorder. Little knowledge of the demonstrated organic damage and deficits associated with FAS has made it into the legal system. However, the organic brain damage caused by prenatal alcohol exposure often does limit a person's ability to form intent and understand behavioral consequences. It is this reality that needs to be detailed in an evaluation and clearly communicated to the court.

Capacity is legally distinguished from diminished capacity. Capacity is based on age. Children under eight are presumed by law (at least in the State of Washington) to not have mental capacity to commit a crime, thus they cannot be charged with a crime. For children between the ages of eight and twelve, if evidence exists that removes this presumption, they may be sent to trial. If a child between eight and twelve is found to not have capacity, the case is dismissed.

FAS evaluations, capacity and diminished capacity. Determination of both capacity and diminished capacity require an evaluation by a qualified expert. Diagnoses of Fetal Alcohol Syndrome are made by specially trained physicians. It is very rare that the expert who can make a diagnosis of FAS is also qualified to make a determination of capacity and/or diminished capacity. However, both of these procedures need to be coordinated and done in conjunction with each other.

If a child under the age of twelve (or slightly older) is referred for a capacity evaluation, a preliminary question must be asked: Was the child exposed to prenatal alcohol? If the child has been prenatally exposed, the next step should be a referral to a physician qualified to make a diagnosis. The psychological/capacity evaluation of a child with FAS should focus on the child's ability to understand cause and effect, to understand the outcome of his/her own behavior, and to articulate abstract concepts. During an evaluation, it should be kept in mind that children with FAS often appear chatty and more capable than they actually are. This can lead evaluators to assume that a child with FAS has the capacity to understand right and wrong and the legal process when, in actuality, the child is simply guessing and giving an answer he/she thinks the evaluator wants.

In the case of diminished capacity, the issue is one of "intent, of motivation." While many people with FAS have IQ scores suggesting an apparent ability to understand cause and effect, this needs to be carefully examined and detailed in any evaluation. Many people with FAS do not have such an understanding and do not have the ability to form intent. However, the cognitive deficits often present in people with FAS are frequently misunderstood and these people are *not* found to have diminished capacity.

Evaluations for people with FAS to determine capacity and diminished capacity need to include an IQ test focusing on abstracting abilities, verbal skills, and the ability to connect cause and effect. Personality tests and clinical interviews focusing on psychiatric functioning should be coupled with intellectual tests and past behavior to fully determine intent. Again, given that many people with FAS look more functional than is the case, care should be taken to review enough records, gain collateral information, and to administer enough tests to provide validation of all deficits. A diagnosis of FAS, in and of itself, is not enough to provide this validation.

Competency

Often the first step when a person with FAS is arrested, charged, and entered into the legal system is a determination of the person's competency to stand trial. Both of the youths in the following vignettes were prenatally exposed to alcohol and both were diagnosed with Fetal Alcohol Syndrome. However, one was found incompetent to stand trial and the charges were dropped, and one was found competent. These decisions were not based solely on IQ but on a variety of factors. This section is intended to present an overview of the competency issue and its connection with Fetal Alcohol Syndrome. It is intended to provoke thought but, by no means, is it the final word on the subject. However, given how many people with FAS already appear to be in or entering the legal system, it is a critical issue to explore.

Tony H. was a seventeen-year-old youth of Hispanic descent who was referred by his attorney and social worker for a psychological evaluation to determine his competency to stand trial on charges of assault. He was accused of assaulting his mother, a woman known to have used alcohol and other substances during her pregnancy. Tony had been in and out of his mother's home and was currently living periodically with one of his older siblings, but mostly he had been living on the street. Tony was a short, slender youth who looked several years younger than his chronological age. He had small eyes, a long, smooth philtrum, mild ptosis and strabismus, and a pattern of behavior consistent with prenatal alcohol exposure.

Tony's IQ scores were in the low-average range but his adaptive behavior skills were much lower than average. His academic achievement scores were in the third to fourth grade range. Tony showed a rudimentary understanding of the charges against him and the legal process. He was able to recount what had lead to the assault charges and what had been inappropriate about his behavior. On this basis, coupled with his IQ scores, past record, and the results of the clinical interview, Tony was found competent to stand trial.

Frankie was a fourteen-year-old boy of Asian/Caucasian/Native American descent who was referred for testing by his probation officer and social worker to determine his competency to stand trial on burglary charges. He lived with his mother, step-father, and two younger half-siblings. He had gone into several houses on his street and taken a variety of items. He then took these items home to his mother and told her how he and his friends had "found" them. His mother called the police and Frankie was charged with 2nd degree burglary. He had not had any previous legal problems.

Frankie was a very small, slender child who appeared closer to ten than fourteen. He had small, wide-spread eyes, a long, smooth philtrum, a flattened midface, marked ptosis, mild strabismus, and noticeably rotated ears. His mother acknowledged consuming at least a fifth of vodka almost every day during her pregnancy. Frankie was born six weeks premature and weighed only three pounds at birth.

Frankie's IQ scores were in the mildly mentally retarded range. His achievement scores for reading, spelling, and arithmetic were all below the third grade level. His adaptive behavior scores were in the 40th percentile. He was not able to articulate what the charges against him were nor could he explain why he was in court. The evaluator found him incompetent to stand trial.

A second evaluation was conducted by a psychologist hired by the State. This psychologist, and later the judge, found Frankie competent. As a result of the court's finding, Frankie entered a plea of guilty rather than waiting for a trial. When the judge attempted to enter the plea, he was required to interview Frankie. He found Frankie was unable to answer even rudimentary questions regarding the legal process or charges against him. The judge reversed himself, found Frankie incompetent, and the charges were dropped.

Competency involves a person's ability to understand the charges against him/her and the legal process, and to aid his/her attorney in the defense in a reasonable fashion. If a person is found incompetent to stand trial, the case is dismissed. Competency is different from capacity. Competency involves a person's ability to understand the legal system; capacity involves a person's ability to form the intent to commit a crime.

A competency evaluation should include an intelligence test, a measure of social interaction style and social competency, projective tests that look at emotional functioning, and a screening test for possible organic damage. In addition, police reports, victim's statements, past psychological evaluations, past probation reports, school reports, and any other background information should be gathered and reviewed prior to completing and writing up the evaluation.

The clinical interview should be used to provide collaboration for test results and background information. A person with FAS, as noted, often appears able to comprehend "yes" or "no" questions and to respond in a semi-appropriate fashion. If interview questions are not phrased in such a way as to demonstrate the person's full functioning level, he/she may be found competent when, in reality, he/she is not. Closed-ended questions (Who is your attorney? Who is the judge? Do you understand that you are on trial?) should be avoided. Closed-ended questions do not allow the person to articulate his/her level of comprehension nor do responses to these questions demonstrate the person's ability to help the attorney in a reasonable fashion. Competency is not simply a matter of "yes" or "no" responding. People with FAS can respond with correct "yes" or "no" answers; what is lacking is a deeper understanding of the consequences of behavior and all possible outcomes.

The evaluator should ask open-ended questions that test whether the patient can comprehend, plan, and understand social rules and expectations. When questioning the person with FAS to help determine competency, questions should be phrased to elicit as much information as possible, for example, What are the charges against you? What do these mean? Why are you going to court? What is your attorney's job? What does the prosecutor do? What does the judge do? What will happen when you go to court? Another difficulty is that, when asked open-ended questions, people with FAS may give conflicting stories and be seen as lying rather than the actuality of having poor memory, recall, and articulation skills.

Decline

Larry G. was a seventeen-year-old single male of Native American descent who was referred for an evaluation to determine if he should be retained in the juvenile justice system or declined into the adult correctional system. Larry had been charged with attempted and first degree murder. He had been involved in a gang fight and had fired a pistol three times, killing one youth and paralyzing another.

Larry was the third of four children born to his mother by different fathers. Larry's family background was characterized by chaos, neglect, abuse, and little support or structure. Larry's father was deceased and his mother appeared to have little ability to manage her son's life or take adequate care of him. His mother estimated drinking a fifth of vodka and a six-pack of beer every day during her pregnancy.

Larry dropped out of school in the ninth grade. Although he had been in regular classes, he was reported to have academic and behavioral (fighting, swearing, and truancy) problems in school. Shortly before his arrest on the current charges, he had been expelled from school for carrying a concealed weapon. Larry had joined a gang when he was about twelve but described his involvement in gang activity as minimal. He had several previous legal charges ranging from taking a motor vehicle without permission to assault in the first degree. The severity and frequency of his criminal activities had been escalating prior to the shooting incident. Larry had recently begun to use and abuse a wide variety of substances including alcohol, cocaine, crack cocaine, LSD, and marijuana. He claimed to have been moderately successful at selling drugs.

Larry's IQ scores were in the average range. However, his adaptive behavior skills test scores and academic achievement test scores were thirty to forty points below his IQ scores, placing him in the lowest one percent of the population. These scores are consistent with what is frequently seen in children who have been prenatally exposed to alcohol.

Larry was referred for an FAS diagnostic evaluation. Based on the physical examination (facial characteristics), prenatal history, and CNS damage, manifested in his behavior and learning deficits, Larry was given a diagnosis of FAS.

Despite Larry's age and his FAS diagnosis, Larry was tried as an adult rather than as a juvenile. Larry's increasing frequency and severity of antisocial behavior, the lack of community and family support systems, his high risk of reoffending, and the continuing risk *he presented to the community all factored into the judge's decision to try Larry as an adult. He was ultimately charged and convicted of second degree murder. He received a sentence of 21 years in medium to maximum security. He is currently serving out his term in an adult facility.*

Brian H. was a thirteen-year-old male of mixed African American/Caucasian descent. He was referred for testing by his probation officer for an evaluation to determine his level of intellectual and social functioning. Brian, despite his young age, had a long history of criminal behavior. His probation officer was concerned about his risk to reoffend and was also seeking help in making treatment and residential decisions.

Brian was the youngest of three children born to an alcoholic mother. He was removed from his mother's care due to neglect. It is not clear if he was physically or sexually abused; however, this was a concern as Brian was beginning to act out in a sexually inappropriate fashion. Brian's home life was described as chaotic, unstable, and dangerous. By the age of thirteen, he had already been charged with robbery, assault, theft, and repeated probation violations.

Brian was referred for an FAS diagnostic evaluation and received a diagnosis of FAS. It was strongly suggested that Brian be placed in either a structured residential program or therapeutic foster home. In addition, vocational training and learning that was based on visual skills was recommended. These services were not implemented for reasons that remain unclear. A presentencing officer later stated, in somewhat ironic fashion, "Brian simply slipped through the service cracks." Brian continued to roam from home to home and to be out on the street. His gang involvement increased. Sadly to say, fourteen months after the first psychological evaluation, Brian shot and killed another youth in a fight.

There was significant discussion, given that Brian was only fourteen, as to whether he should be declined or retained in the juvenile system. His increasing level of dangerous behavior and concerns over his risk to reoffend led to him being declined into the adult system. Brian was charged with, and convicted of, second degree assault and murder. He was sentenced to fifteen years and is currently serving his sentence in a juvenile maximum security facility. He will be transferred to an adult facility at either age 18 or 21.

The decision to try an offender as a juvenile or as an adult is made at a decline hearing. The primary issue in a decline hearing is whether a juvenile should be *retained* in the juvenile system or *declined* into the adult system. Decisions to decline are based on evaluations performed by a mental health professional such as a psychologist or psychiatrist. The evaluating professional makes the determination by assessing the family background, the educational and achievement level, and the previous history in the juvenile justice system of the alleged offender. Community resources and the possibility of reintegration into the community also are considered. A decision to decline must be made with serious thought because an adolescent once held to adult standards, will forever be treated as an adult.

Specifically, the decision to decline an individual into the adult system or remand the individual in the juvenile system is based on several factors. These include the following:

1. Period of Incarceration
   a. A judge will weigh differences in sentencing and periods of incarceration between the adult and juvenile systems. The juvenile system's maximum period of incarceration is commitment to age 21 or no longer than the adult maximum. The standard range in the adult system generally carries a longer period of incarceration.

2. "Kent" Criteria ("yes" responses to the following questions increase the potential for a juvenile to be declined, although any one factor by itself *can* result in a decline)
   a. Was the alleged offense a serious offense to the community? Does the community require protection?
   b. Was the alleged offense committed in an aggressive, violent, premeditated or willful manner?
   c. Was the alleged offense against another person or persons? Did anyone get injured?
   d. Does the prosecutor have a good chance of winning the case?
   e. Are any of the juvenile's associates adults charged with a crime? Will it be more cost effective and efficient to try everyone together as adults?
   f. Is the juvenile sufficiently sophisticated and mature, considering his home, environmental situation, emotional attitude, and pattern of living?
   g. Does the juvenile have a record or previous history of contacts with the law, juvenile courts and other jurisdictions, prior to periods of probation or prior commitments to juvenile institutions?

h. Rehabilitation — Is it unlikely that the juvenile can be reasonably rehabilitated by use of procedures, services, and facilities available to the juvenile court?

The possibility for successful rehabilitation often is a primary consideration in determining whether or not to decline a juvenile. In many cases, the possibility for successful rehabilitation involves the offender's ability to learn from his/her mistakes and to avoid making the same poor decisions or displaying the same impulsive behavior that led to problems in the first place. Because of the brain damage associated with FAS, "true" rehabilitation, specifically the ability to learn from past behavior and mistakes, often is not possible for people with FAS.

The impact of FAS on meeting the Kent criteria for decline is something that usually is not taken into account in the juvenile justice system. For example, protection of the community is primary and must be considered. However, many times, if the crime is not of a violent and/or repetitive nature, a structured residential placement, with vocational training and behavioral management programs, can achieve the same end as can incarceration.

With a person with FAS, it also is important that the safety of the *offender* be taken into account. Many people with FAS have poor social skills and a high level of impulsivity. Their immaturity puts them at risk for problems both within and without correctional facilities. For this reason, it is often more appropriate to have the offender housed in a juvenile facility where the emphasis is on treatment rather than on punishment.

The issue of sophistication and maturity is another component of the Kent criteria that should be taken into consideration when determining the appropriateness of decline. As mentioned above, many people with FAS are much less insightful than their chronological age suggests. They do not, despite attempts at insight therapy or other interventions, increase their skills in this area. It is important that the psychological evaluation assess this area. This should be a primary concern before the decision to decline is made.

Yet another area of concern when making a decline determination is the criminal record and previous history of the juvenile. As in the case studies presented at the start of this section, it is common for juvenile offenders with FAS to have many offenses on their records. Often, the juvenile's rate of offending increases with the lessening of supervision. In the second example, Brian had little structure or supervision. Later information strongly suggested that his mother may have FAS herself.

The Kent criteria suggests looking at the juvenile's associates. People with FAS are easily influenced, good followers, and freely manipulated. They are the ones who would jump off the proverbial bridge if asked to do so by a friend. Given these factors, it is crucial that the juvenile with FAS be evaluated separately from his peers.

Both young men described at the beginning of this section, sad to say, met many of the criteria that led to decline decisions. Both came from chaotic environments, had serious histories of criminal behaviors, had serious difficulties in school, had long histories of acting out behavior, and were at high risk to reoffend.

Additional suggestions. Two additional suggestions for decline evaluations could help other young offenders with FAS achieve more appropriate placements in the future.

First, an assessment of the family history and present environment should be made. This assessment will include parental or caregiver resources such as finances, emotional stability, ability to participate in decision-making, and ability to provide positive, consistent, and nurturing structure. These factors will play a crucial role in whether preventive steps can be taken to keep the youth in the community or if a more restrictive environment will be needed.

Second, if the youth is in an offending pattern, the factors that are either supportive or possibly disruptive of this pattern should be assessed. The youth's skills and community resources that support his/her skills need to be accessed and incorporated into a positive support system. This can be accomplished by a team approach, which could include

a. An initial diagnosis by a dysmorphologist or other qualified expert in the diagnosis of birth defects;
b. Consultation with an educational specialist, psychologist, behavioral management specialist, court advocate (e.g., attorney), and social worker;
c. Close consultation with the parent, caregiver, or advocate of the patient; and
d. Careful consideration of the needs and wishes of the patient.

This evaluation should, ideally, occur prior to any court proceedings and in conjunction with the psychological evaluation. The team approach can assess all of the factors listed under the Kent criteria and, hopefully, provide enough data to make choices that will truly benefit the needs of the patient, the family, the community, and society.

The diagnosis of FAS, alone, is not enough to rule against a decline decision. However, FAS and its impact on brain functioning and behavior must be taken into account when making such a decision regarding an affected person. The team approach detailed above can be an invaluable tool in collecting needed data to help the court make the best, most appropriate, and most humane determination.

An Alternative Outcome: A Success Story

Kattina was a sixteen-year-old, single female of Hispanic/Filipino descent. She was the only child born to a mother who was thirteen years old at the time of Kattina's birth. Kattina's mother acknowledged consuming up to 12 beers or more per day. Kattina's biological father was unknown.

Kattina had been diagnosed with Fetal Alcohol Syndrome when she was eight. Her mother had relinquished her to foster care due to her alcoholism and transient lifestyle. When Kattina was fifteen, she was living on the street, using and dealing drugs, and involved in prostitution. She joined a gang and ended up in an altercation where she repeatedly stabbed another young woman.

Kattina was referred for a decline evaluation. Her IQ score was 102, but her academic achievement scores indicated that she was at the third grade level in reading, spelling, and arithmetic. Her adaptive behavior skills corresponded to average scores of eight-year-olds. Kattina demonstrated little common sense, a high level of impulsive behavior, almost no understanding of cause and effect, and a seeming inability to understand the seriousness of her crime.

She had no family support, having run away from every one of many foster placements. She had not attended school on a regular basis for two years. However, her only previous criminal history had been two charges of taking a motor vehicle without permission and one charge of prostitution.

Given the above information, the evaluator recommended retention in the juvenile system, with the court to retain jurisdiction in the juvenile system. However, because of aggravating factors, she was sentenced to a longer term than might have been usual for her crime, a condition legally known as a "Manifest Injustice." Kattina was given a sentence of 102 weeks in a juvenile facility and then was put on a "tight" and closely monitored probation for three years following her release.

Part of her probation was to attend school, get a job for after school, attend weekly therapy sessions, and attend drug and alcohol treatment on an out-patient basis. These are common conditions of juvenile probation which are not always followed. In Kattina's case, three critical events happened that lead to a positive outcome.

The first event was a meeting held just prior to Kattina's decline hearing. The meeting was attended by the probation officer, defense attorney, social worker, prosecutor, evaluating psychologist, presiding judge, and Kattina. Kattina's medical, psychosocial, and school records all were carefully examined. It was decided to let Kattina plead guilty to the assault charge with the provision of the "Manifest Injustice." The judge educated himself about FAS and agreed to the conditions listed above. However, it was also understood that, should Kattina reoffend upon her release, she would be tried as an adult on any charges.

The second event was her biological mother's entrance into a shelter and request for drug and alcohol treatment. The public health nurse running the shelter suspected that Kattina's mother had FAS. This turned out to be the case and her mother was placed on Social Security and given a protective payee, subsidized housing, and vocational training. She also entered a long-term treatment program that offered life skills along with vocational training. Kattina's mother is still involved in this program. Kattina and her mother have reconnected and are attending therapy sessions together.

The third event that occurred was Kattina's development of a relationship with the adoptive parents of another young girl while in the juvenile facility. These parents decided to ask if they could foster Kattina as part of her parole. The parents had worked with special needs children before, including several with FAS, and were actively involved in a community support group. The Court allowed this placement and, as of today, with tight supervision and constant structure, Kattina is living with her foster parents and is doing well. The parents reported that she is not using drugs and her truancy and seriously assaultive behavior have stopped.

Kattina has become sexually active again and this is of some concern. Kattina, so far, has tested negative for HIV but has had several bouts of venereal warts, chlamydia, and gonorrhea. She has difficulty, despite her normal IQ, truly comprehending things such as "safe sex" and personal boundaries. However, the therapy and other aspects of her probation have been strictly adhered to by her foster family. In addition, Kattina has connected with her biological mother and is attending some therapy sessions with her. Art therapy and behavioral management rather than insight have been the primary tools of this therapy.

Kattina is no longer in regular school courses. She is in a community-based vocational training program for computer skills and has a part-time job where she earns a salary for using these skills. She still has periods of angry outbursts but these are lessening. Her family *has a schedule written out and posted in several spots around the house. This has made it easier for Kattina to understand expectations and boundaries.*

Kattina's story has not yet ended. What has made the difference for Kattina was that the juvenile justice system allowed enough flexibility for Kattina's needs to be met in an unusual fashion and that Kattina had the good fortune to find foster parents who understood FAS and who would advocate for their child. She will need this type of support for the rest of her life. The question is: Where will such future support come from? Hopefully, the Courts will take more time, hold pretrial meetings, and work together to support and aid these children, not just to punish and warehouse them.

FAS: Preventing and Treating Sexual Deviancy

Natalie Novick

According to recent research (see chapter by Streissguth, Barr, Kogan, & Bookstein), inappropriate sexual behavior (ISB) is one of the most prevalent secondary disabilities of Fetal Alcohol Syndrome (FAS) and Fetal Alcohol Effects (FAE). ISB is defined as any compulsive and problematic sexual behavior or any behavior that results in sentencing of an individual for sexual offender treatment. For children between the ages of six and eleven, ISB ranks second in prevalence among secondary disabilities after mental health problems. For adolescents between 12 and 20, ISB ranks fourth after mental health problems, disrupted school experience, and trouble with the law. For adults between the ages of 21 and 51, ISB ranks fifth, following confinement (i.e., imprisonment) in addition to the four secondary disabilities previously mentioned.

Evaluaters and treaters of individuals who have been charged with sexual crimes traditionally have not acknowledged the role of FAS or FAE in criminal behavior. Regardless of a person's ability to understand the nature of his/her actions and the consequences of that behavior, the sexual offender with FAS/FAE is not treated any differently than is an offender without such a diagnosis. The result of this lack of differentiation has been inaccurate assessment, improper treatment, and inappropriate incarceration. The following case study presents an illustration of how the approach to evaluation and treatment for sexual offenders with FAS can accommodate the special needs of these individuals. Following the case study is a separate section on how parents of children who are beginning to engage in inappropriate sexual touching can identify this problem and respond with techniques aimed at preventing criminal conduct.

Case Study

Joey* was 36 when I first met him. He had been referred by his attorney after being charged with two counts of Rape of a Child in

*Names and details have been changed to maintain client confidentiality.

the Third Degree. These charges stemmed from incidents in 1994 involving a young boy named Kevin who was 14 years old at the time. The two reportedly had known each other for about three years prior to the sexual abuse. They had met through mutual friends, who were about Kevin's age. Joey did not have any friends his own age; instead, he hung out with teenage boys, who accepted him in a peripheral way but also teased and taunted him because he was not very quick-witted. According to Joey, he and Kevin were "close friends." Joey would take Kevin to restaurants and buy him gifts. According to Kevin, who later gave a victim statement to police, he and Joey were "acquaintances," even though they saw each other almost every day.

Joey had worked in his father's successful recreational vehicle (RV) business for years as a detailer (i.e., he washed and cleaned RVs) but kept having difficulty getting along with some of his father's supervisors. As the son of the company's owner, Joey expected to be eventually promoted to a prestigious management position within the company and constantly was frustrated with his lack of progress. The supervisors, in turn, were frustrated with having to accommodate the son of the owner, who had to be told over and over how to do basic tasks that he had previously done many times. Joey occasionally would quit when he became frustrated with the "lack of respect" from these supervisors and find alternative work as a dishwasher or short-order cook. After a few days or weeks in another job, he would return to the dealership and begin detailing cars again.

On the day of the first incident of sexual molestation, Joey had quit working for his father's company and was planning to drive to another city to look for employment. He asked Kevin to accompany him, and the two drove off together. Once in a new city, Joey got them a room in a motel. According to Kevin, once in the room, Joey started becoming sexually aggressive with him. Joey tried several different sexual behaviors with Kevin, including anal intercourse. Kevin told police later that he kept resisting these advances. Finally, Joey fell asleep, and the two returned home the next day without any further incident.

Following this first incident of sexual abuse, there were two other occasions when Joey attempted to sexually molest Kevin. The third, and final, occasion took place in Joey's truck parked outside the home of Kevin's family. Kevin allowed Joey to sexually touch him this third time, and the two were engaged in sexual activity when Kevin's family came outside and discovered them together in the truck. Kevin's family phoned the police, and Joey was arrested and charged.

When I first met Joey for his psychosexual evaluation, he was in denial about what he had done and blamed Kevin for the sexual molestation. As we talked, he began to reveal details about his childhood that suggested he was likely fetal alcohol impaired. According to his report, his adoptive parents found out several years after he had been adopted that his biological mother had been an alcoholic and had been actively drinking throughout her pregnancy. The agency which had sponsored the adoption had not informed them of this at the time of the adoption.

The initial step in Joey's psychosexual evaluation was to obtain a complete history from him, including childhood experiences, relationship history, and sexual history. Joey talked easily about his childhood, and responded positively to my attention and interest in him. He revealed that his childhood was very difficult, and his adoptive parents, who did not know about FAS or about Joey's likely diagnosis, were overwhelmed by his problems. Joey told me, "I was not like a normal kid. I was slow. I still am in a way. I became scared of everyone because kids teased me. I got beat up by older boys every day at school. I learned you just had to do whatever they told you to do." Joey reported that his adoptive parents would fight over how to raise him. They could not figure out why he had so many behavioral problems (e.g., stealing, lying, truancy, aggressive behavior, inappropriate touching of other children), and why their younger son, who was also adopted, was relatively easy to raise.

Joey described his school experience in negative terms, "School was a joke. I was in 'special ed' (special education) in the first grade. I was stuck in this class with rowdy kids who did not care about learning. So, I never learned anything. To this day, I have not learned how to multiple or divide. I can read, but I can not spell. I spent all my elementary school years in special ed. The other kids called us Edders. No matter how much I asked, my mother would not get me out of special ed." Similarly to the way he blamed his victim for the sexual abuse, Joey had a tendency to blame his mother for his childhood problems. One of the characteristics I have observed in sexual offense clients with suspected fetal alcohol impairment is a diminished ability to take personal responsibility for their behavior. This makes it more difficult for them to become motivated in treatment to change their behavior.

The rest of Joey's history was similar. He got into drugs as an adolescent and acted out with his peers in order to be accepted. However, he never was accepted as part of the group and finally dropped out of school in the 11th grade to begin working full-time for his father's business. Socially, he was very shy with girls his own age and reported no dating and very limited social involvement with same-age females throughout his teen and adult years. He had had his first sexual encounter at the age of 10 when he was molested by a boy two years older than he was. When he was 21, he had his first and only sexual experience with a young woman who was 19, whom he had met while talking on the CB radio. When he was in his 20's, he had two other experiences with women which did not result in sexual intimacy because the women quickly became disillusioned with him. As a result of his limited sexual experience, he felt inadequate with women his own age.

The evaluation process for this client conformed to the standards in Washington State, although more time than is usual was spent on his family history and childhood behavior in order to determine if he met criteria for FAS. He was interviewed extensively, and his adoptive parents also were interviewed. The latter typically is not done in sexual offense evaluations, but, in the case of a possible FAS diagnosis, which would affect the recommendations, this was considered essential. In addition to interviews, Joey was administered two personality tests and a sexual history questionnaire. He was given assistance in completing these tests, which revealed a passive-aggressive character, low self-esteem, need for attention, and tendency to act out impulsively. He also was administered an IQ test, which revealed an intellectual ability in the low average range.

Two physiological tests, the polygraph and plethysmograph, were included in the test battery that was administered to Joey. He passed the polygraph exam, which included questions that asked if he had ever sexually touched any other minor, male or female, other than Kevin. Joey responded, "No." The second physiological test was a penile plethysmograph. This test measures sexual arousal to a variety of slides, audio tapes, and videotapes that depict the full range of sexual behavior, including sexual behavior between adult males and young boys Kevin's age. Joey's results were interesting. His arousal to adult and minor females barely was significant. His arousal to adult males and males between the ages of 15 and 18 was insignificant. However, his arousal to boys between 12 and 14 was in the high moderate range. His arousal to boys between 8 and 11 was in the low moderate range. His arousal to boys between 4 and 7 was in the mild range. All this suggested a sexually deviant arousal pattern that would have to be addressed with arousal reconditioning techniques in treatment.

Finally, Joey was asked to comment on his victim's statements as they appeared in the police report. He began the evaluation by denying any responsibility for what had occurred. To him, Kevin was the

aggressor, and he was the victim. However, by the end of the evaluation, he was beginning to acknowledge that, as the adult, he was the
one who was responsible. This enabled me to recommend treatment
for this client. At sentencing, the judge was interested in Joey's
possible diagnosis of FAS and his ability to learn and benefit from
treatment given this diagnosis. I told him that individuals with FAS
or developmental disabilities usually did very poorly in prison. They
are quickly targeted as victims and often sexually abused themselves.
They emerge from their prison experience with many more problems
than they had going in, one of these problems being sexual behavior
that is out of control.

Fortunately, Joey received treatment in lieu of a prison sentence
and began a three year cognitive-behavioral program that was
designed to teach clients how to control their behavior by controlling their thoughts and feelings. He is now in the process of learning
about his sexual offense cycle. He is learning that negative core
beliefs about himself and unhealthy ways of coping with stress
contributed to his sexual acting out, as well as did what we call
"impaired thinking." An example of impaired thinking for Joey was
his tendency to think of Kevin as an equal in terms of responsibility
for sexual behavior.

Joey is in his second year of treatment now and has just
completed sexual arousal reconditioning, which pairs aversive
stimuli with deviant sexual scenarios. This process is designed to
eliminate deviant arousal. He has also been through an assignment
that required him to put himself in the role of his victim and write
his victim a letter of apology. This has been a particularly difficult
assignment for Joey because he has a problem with concepts and
abstract thinking. However, what was effective for him was bringing
in an adult victim of childhood sexual abuse, who gave Joey's group
a first-hand account of what it felt like to be molested as a young boy
by an adult male. Currently, Joey is receiving anger management
training and is about to begin a section on social skills development,
which for him is very much needed and will support the process of
building his self-esteem and self-confidence with adult women.

Joey has not reoffended since starting treatment, which is in part
due to the support he is receiving from both his mother (with whom
he currently lives) and from other members of his group. For the first
time in his life, he feels accepted and a part of a group. He seems
motivated to control his behavior, but the difficult time will come
when treatment is finished, and he is on his own. Like other clients
with fetal alcohol impairments and developmental disabilities,
compliance with treatment — with all the structure we build into the

process — is relatively easy compared to life outside of treatment, where there are no rules, no restrictions, and no one watching over the client.

In order to prevent re-offense among offenders with FAS, some form of treatment aftercare and monitoring on a long-term basis is essential. Another critical need for such individuals is a structured, supportive living environment both during and after treatment. At present, there are few resources that offer such an environment. Group homes are one alternative, particularly for individuals who need 24-hour supervision. For individuals who are somewhat self-sufficient, independent living situations involving frequent and regular assistance from a skilled counselor or advisor may be appropriate. Without such ancillary resources, no matter how good the treatment program is or how motivated the client is while in treatment, prognosis is poor. Aftercare support must be available, perhaps for many years, in order to sustain the motivation and the positive behavior changes that have been made.

What is even more effective than a strong treatment and aftercare response, however, is preventive work. Joey's legal problems could have been avoided if his parents had known about his diagnosis from the beginning and been able to take steps to minimize the problems he was likely to have as a result of his impairments. In particular, had they known what to expect and look for in his behavior and how to address incipient problems before they had a chance to escalate into illegal behavior, Joey's life might have taken a more positive direction.

Advice to Parents

The challenge for parents of children with FAS/FAE who have begun to engage in inappropriate touching of other children is to stop the behaviors before they reach the level of becoming criminal offenses. Instruction for such children must be very basic and must clearly delineate consequences for failure to follow "rules" regarding social conduct. The objective is absolute clarity and understanding on the part of the child, who — despite difficulty with abstract thinking — must know key concepts that relate to ISB prevention and how these concepts relate to him or her personally.

The concept of "rules" is most important. In therapy, I ask the child if he has any rules at home or at school, and we begin by talking about those rules. I ask him what makes something a rule (e.g., expectation and requirements of parents and teachers), why it is good to follow the rules, what happens if you do not follow the rules. I ask what would happen if there were no rules. For example, what would it be like to live in a house where there were no rules? What would it be like to go to a school where there were no rules? The conclusion we want the child to arrive at is that rules keep us safe.

Other key concepts include boundary (e.g., dividing line, physical space between people, where one leaves off and another begins), private places (e.g., genital areas, breasts, buttocks), sexual (e.g., people touching each other in private places, wanting to touch somebody who is attractive), physical (e.g., something to do with someone's body, something that can be seen/felt/touched), social (e.g., being with other people, talking and doing things with other people), and emotional (e.g., feelings such as anger, sadness, happiness, frustration, jealousy, love, attraction).

Once the child understands the meanings of the key words, we begin to work on using these words conceptually. We begin first with boundaries, or sets of rules about how to act with other people. Ask the child: How close do you get to someone else? When you are working near somebody, how close do you get? When do you touch somebody else? When is it not okay to touch somebody? How do you touch someone? What kinds of touching are okay in what situations? Once a child has a basic understanding of the concepts, we begin to differentiate different kinds of boundaries.

For example, with regard to physical boundaries, the objective is to have the child understand that he or she touches someone else *only with permission*. To teach the child this concept, ask the following questions:

> *Who can touch you and whom can you touch?*
> *When is it okay for you to touch someone or for them to touch you?*
> *How close do you sit or stand to people? (personal space)*
> *When do you make eye contact?*
> *How close do you get to people in elevators?*
> *How close do you get to people while waiting in lines?*

To teach a child that sexual touching is only allowed between grown-ups, ask the following questions:

> *Whom do you let touch you in a sexual way?*
> *Whom is it okay for you to touch in a sexual way?*
> *Who can see you with your clothes off?*
> *When is it okay to touch somebody's private places?*
> *What do you do if you want to touch someone's private places?*

To protect the child from being victimized, ask the following questions:

With whom is it okay to talk?
Is it ever okay to talk to strangers?
What do you do when a stranger starts talking to you?
What do you do if a stranger touches you in a private place?
When is it okay to talk to others?
With whom do you do things/socialize?

Finally, in order to teach the child how to talk about his/her feelings with respect to sexual issues, ask the following questions:

Who controls your feelings?
How do you control your feelings?
Do you have a right to talk about your feelings?
When is it okay/not okay to talk about feelings?
With whom should you talk about your feelings?

Once the child understands the key words and the concepts, we begin to apply these ideas with vignettes and examples relevant to the child's experience:

Example 1

Kathy has very poor personal boundaries. Sometimes, she stares at people she does not know. Other times, she bumps into people in the lunch line at school. Kathy wants to be best friends with Sarah. She watches Sarah all the time at school. One day, at recess, she sees Sarah eating a snack on a bench in the play area. Kathy walks over to her and sits down very close. Sarah says "hi" to Kathy and moves farther away on the bench. Kathy is happy that Sarah said "hi." She watches Sarah eat for a minute and thinks that she is very pretty. She notices that Sarah's hair shines and sparkles in the sunlight. She reaches out her hand and touches Sarah's hair. Sarah jumps up, grabs her lunch, and walks away. *Ask the child: How did Kathy break the NO TOUCHING WITHOUT PERMISSION rule? What was Sarah probably thinking at the time? How should Kathy have behaved?*

Example 2

Michael is nine years old and is best friends with Danny, who is six. They play together all the time. Lately, Michael has begun to rough-house with Danny. He hides in Danny's closet when Danny leaves his room, and when Danny returns,

Michael jumps out and tackles him to the ground. One day, Michael tackles Danny, and the two are rolling around laughing on the floor. Michael starts tickling Danny on the side of his body. Then, he tickles him in his private area. Danny keeps laughing, so Michael thinks it is okay to keep tickling him in his private area. *How did Michael break the NO SEXUAL TOUCHING UNTIL YOU ARE GROWN UP rule? What was Danny probably thinking? What might Danny do after Michael touched him? Did Michael break any other rules?*

Parents of a fetal alcohol impaired child who has not yet begun to explore his or her sexuality have an advantage. The best way to prevent inappropriate sexual touching is to give the child guidelines and coping skills he or she can use when faced with a desire to make physical contact with another person. Contact the local school district or public library to obtain information used in the sex education curriculum and modify that information to make it more appropriate for the fetal alcohol-impaired child. The therapeutic approach described above also can be modified to fit the needs and learning ability of a child in question. Since children often begin sexual exploration by the age of nine or ten, parents should begin the process of in-home sex education while their child is in elementary school. In-home instruction should continue as the child reaches junior and senior high school, and parents can facilitate this process by remaining in contact with teaching personnel responsible for in-school sex education.

Parents of children with FAS/FAE who have already begun to engage in sexual touching should contact a therapist specialized in FAS/FAE, child psychology, or developmental psychology for assistance. Make sure that the therapists who are being considered have the appropriate training and experience to work with children on sexual issues. The preferred mode of treatment for such children is cognitive-behavioral therapy, which tends to be far more concrete and directive than other kinds of therapy. Other resources that might be helpful in such situations include local school districts (special education divisions, school counseling services), local and state agencies that deal with children's services and developmental disabilities, the National Council on Disability (202-272-2004), and the National Organization on Fetal Alcohol Syndrome (800-666-6327).

Parent Advocacy in FAS Public Policy Change

Jocie DeVries with Ann Waller

In 1990, my husband and I discovered, after 16 harrowing years, that the origin of trauma for our adopted son's unusual brain damage was heavy prenatal alcohol exposure. The most alarming factor to us was not that Fetal Alcohol Syndrome (FAS) was a life-long disability; what alarmed us most was that the professionals to whom we went for help — counselors, school teachers, social workers, psychiatrists, medical doctors, police, probation officers, attorneys and judges — were unable to recognize clients with FAS on their caseloads.

This chapter focuses on the efforts of parents working together out of common experience and desperation. Our driving goal originally was, and still is, to improve the lives of individuals with FAS and their families. While pursuing this goal, we found ourselves involved in a concerted effort to change public policy in Washington State. This process began, for us, in 1990 when FAS was an obscure disability in public policy circles and proceeds to 1996 when Governor Lowry appropriated money from the state emergency fund to support recovering birth mothers of children with FAS. I will share methods we used to improve the lives of children with FAS and their families. It is my goal to help parents and professionals:

- search for effective avenues to educate others about the dangers of prenatal alcohol exposure,

- utilize their own talents, skills, financial resources, and personal experiences to develop public education and intervention programs, and

- strive to produce public policy that identifies, understands, and cares for individuals with FAS and their families and prevents future generations from having to live with this disability.

Parent Advocacy

The 4-Track Developmental Profile

After the initial shock of learning about FAS subsided, my husband and I were able to develop a physical environment to keep

171

our son, Rusty, and the community safe and healthy. Then we began the search to fulfill his other needs: friends, an education, recreation, mental health, and spiritual guidance. He desired to feel useful, to develop his own talents and skills in order to give back to the community. The more organizations we discovered which provide services to people with disabilities, the more we realized that they were either totally void of information about fetal alcohol exposure or they offered services which were only appropriate for individuals who are mentally retarded. No services existed for individuals, like Rusty, who were disabled by permanent damage to their memory, reasoning, and judgment, despite deceivingly acceptable IQ scores. This search for services was so painful that my husband and I vowed that no other family would have to make this journey alone. As we began to connect with other parents, we discovered that this was a common experience of families who had children with FAS and normal IQ's. To meet this void of services, we needed something other than research papers. Most service providers had read the scientific literature on FAS, but still could not recognize individuals with FAS and a normal IQ. We realized that parents needed a vocabulary and a practical way to describe the needs of their children to the professionals to whom they went for help.

As I frantically searched for ways to describe how FAS had impaired the cognitive process of my child, a loving and persistent friend, Rebecca Bangsund, walked beside me and challenged me. We developed a visual graphic that shows the strengths and weaknesses of each individual with FAS, because the brain of each child is uniquely affected. We discovered that the physical, social, educational, and moral developmental histories of each child could be charted so that parents would be able to communicate the specific strengths and core disability characteristics of their children to appropriate service providers. We called this graphic the 4-Track Developmental Profile.

Advocacy Notebooks

Graphics make it easy to communicate difficult and complicated ideas in a short period of time. I developed a notebook filled with current magazine and newspaper articles, with headlines such as, "Why Can't Kids Tell Right from Wrong?" "Whatever Happened to Ethics?" "Where is the Shame?" My notebook became my "advocacy book." As it evolved, I included more articles about FAS, Rusty's life history, and other resources, making it into a complete presentation, which I updated on a continual basis. I used this notebook when speaking with teachers, social workers, counselors, probation officers, etc. I imitated the methods of reporters by trying to answer the questions which were in the minds of the public and the audiences to whom I spoke about FAS. The notebook became a successful visual aid that any parent could use regardless of their level of experience in advocacy and public speaking. Other families developed their own notebooks to use, and these notebooks have become invaluable in our efforts to educate others. With them we have been able to

- communicate to individual professionals about the unique needs of our children and our families;
- educate various community groups;
- testify at legislative committee hearings; and
- provide television and newspaper reporters, who are searching for human interest stories, with a clear understanding of FAS and how this disability impacts the community and society.

FAS Education

My friend and colleague Vicky McKinney and her husband adopted a child with FAS in 1990. Vicky's three teenage sons recognized that their school's drug awareness program gave young adults no education as to the consequences of drinking during pregnancy, while the pregnancy rate and the rate of alcohol consumption among teens was still rising. The need for FAS education prior to pregnancy became critical to us. In response, we created the program, "Prevention at Its Earliest" — a practical, research-based, FAS prevention program which would appeal to young adults. The program's success, according to teachers, lies in the true-life, traumatic stories of individuals with FAS and their families. The understanding that FAS could permanently disable a child of their own gives teens positive motivation to abstain from drinking alcohol during pregnancy. Vicky also adapted her presentation for adult audiences to give them a practical medical overview of FAS. This evolved into her seminar entitled "FAS 101."

Representation of Birth Mothers

Linda LaFever joined our team. She is the birth mother of 14-year-old Danny, who was the first March of Dimes ambassador for FAS in America. Linda's humility and courage cleared away the cobwebs of ignorance for me regarding the trauma and tragedy of alcohol and other drug addictions. She has confronted the grief and shame of being a birth mother of a child with FAS and transformed these emotions into a strong sense of responsibility to educate others about the unique needs of birth families.

The FAS Adolescent Task Force

The success of the 4-Track Developmental Profile, the Advocacy Notebooks, Linda's representation of birth mothers, and Vicky's basic FAS education prompted us to carefully examine the reasons why these educational approaches were successful. We needed this information to replicate and multiply our advocacy efforts. First, we wanted to form a cohesive group of individuals with the same goals in the fields of FAS education and advocacy. We formed a private non-profit organization which we called The FAS Adolescent Task Force (FAS*ATF) in 1991. The focus of this grassroots group was to attack the misconception that FAS only affects toddlers and preschoolers; most people have no idea how to recognize adolescents and adults with FAS, much less connect their disabilities with the critical trends occurring in our society.

Vicky McKinney, Linda LaFever, and I made our phone numbers available to parents and professionals who wanted FAS information and support. Over the next several years we received crisis calls from over 500 families — birth, foster, adoptive, and step parents. We organized and conducted personal interviews and surveys that gathered crucial data, which indicated commonalities among FAS traits and their impact on family relationships. With this database on family issues, members of the FAS*ATF developed several educational programs, in addition to the three we already had developed. Together, these programs help various professional service providers learn how to recognize clients with Fetal Alcohol Syndrome, show service providers how people with FAS impact their specific service systems and affect their personal and professional success. These programs reveal that Fetal Alcohol Syndrome is an invisible avalanche crashing down and overpowering the resources of their agencies, and give practical suggestions and hope to families and professionals who struggle to get out from under this avalanche.

We have found that a key element in these educational programs is parents educating others by sharing their personal experiences regarding the tragic results of prenatal alcohol exposure on the developing brain of the fetus. Research alone cannot transform public opinion. Effective public policy is built on a well balanced educational program — based on both the science of valid research and the art of skillful parenting. It is critical to provide information and strategies based on practical, experienced-based knowledge. This is the most effective way to reveal the often unidentified traumatic and dramatic impact that Fetal Alcohol Syndrome has on individuals, families, communities and society.

We had to learn to separate our grief and anger from the task of getting appropriate services. We quickly realized that those parents who could tell their stories in a manner that showed respect for their audience were the most effective advocates. When working with policy makers, we tried to remember that they are often busy people who are overworked and underappreciated. We felt it was our job to supply them with valid, up-to-date information on the subject of FAS. We publicized their positive responses to us when given the opportunity. Some of the most amusing and beneficial advice, which we received from a long-term disability advocate, was that when you come up against people who refuse to help your children, "step over the dead bodies and keep going." While this statement could be variously interpreted, we took it to mean that when we encountered professionals who would not help us achieve our goals or who refused to listen to us, we did not let their negative responses deter us. Our aim was to be courteous but assertive about the rights and needs of individuals with FAS and their families. A healthy sense of humor helped, too. With this approach we were far more effective advocates than those who lost their temper and yelled obscenities. When our motives and methods remained pure we did not get sidetracked from our goals.

The FAS Family Resource Institute

As we described to professionals how fetal alcohol exposure had affected our families, we began to identify those individuals within agencies who were willing to listen and who had the necessary personal commitment to families to pursue change. A few professionals wanted to join forces with us. We learned early on that it was important to be alert and flexible because we were finding help in unexpected places.

Our organization matured. We grew into addressing the full spectrum of needs of affected individuals and their families, so we changed our name to reflect our expanded activities. We became the FAS Family Resource Institute (FAS*FRI). The mission of the FAS Family Resource Institute is to help professionals and family members identify, understand and care for individuals disabled by prenatal alcohol exposure and to prevent future generations from having to live with this disability.

Public Policy Change Points

As our children grew older and more difficult to handle, we began to realize we would have to help systems fit services for individuals with FAS into their current programs. This led us and other professionals to analyze each of the systems into which our children fell: education, juvenile and criminal justice, developmental disabilities, child welfare, chemical dependency and mental health. Experiencing setbacks at the entry level of each system forced us to quickly learn that the power to make change and develop appropriate programs was in upper management. As the saying goes, "You do not get what you deserve, you get what you negotiate." We discovered that frontline workers did not have the authority to "negotiate" or change department policy. We realized the necessity of changing public policy.

With the help of our efforts, a number of events transpired in Washington State that are proving to be major change points for the future direction of FAS prevention and intervention in Washington State.

Juvenile Justice

In August of 1991, parents spoke about FAS at the Washington State Council on Crime and Delinquency Conference. Our testimony substantiated the impact fetal alcohol was and is making in the juvenile justice system. For the first time, because of the parents' testimony, the professionals in the audience left feeling depressed and the parents left feeling hopeful. A door was opened to public recognition of FAS as a disability. Later that month, the first parent FAS conference was held at Children's Hospital in Seattle. My presentation of the 4-Track Developmental Profile astonished many parents because they recognized the same lack of moral development in their disabled children. Although each child was affected very differently in the other life domains, the arrested moral development was apparent throughout this population.

Families raising adolescents with FAS across the state mobilized to testify at the statewide Juvenile Justice Hearings in the fall of 1991. At the hearings, we commended agency personnel and legislators for their concern with juvenile offenders, but explained why their good programs were not appropriate treatment for adolescent offenders with FAS. The Secretary of the Department of Social and Health Services, a member of the Juvenile Justice Panel, heard our testimony and scheduled FAS training for agency personnel.

Senator Pam Roach and Representative June Leonard called a joint hearing of the House and Senate committees on children and family services in December of 1991, to determine the impact of FAS on state systems. Our experience-based testimony offered insight into the questions of why the juvenile crime rate continued to climb and why FAS prevention programs were critical to the future of the state. After our testimony, state policy makers confirmed our statements that FAS was having a traumatic impact on state systems.

Parents were flooded by a new interest of the media in issues surrounding FAS. It became obvious that we needed to develop appropriate skills in responding to the media to promote fetal alcohol prevention and education, while protecting the privacy of our families. These skills were acquired through media training by the March of Dimes and became an essential piece of our advocacy.

We gave private FAS presentations to Mary Lowry (the First Lady of Washington State), Christine Gregoire (the Attorney General), Judith Billings (the Superintendent of Public Instruction), June Leonard (the Chair of the House of Representatives' Children and Family Services Committee), and Pam Roach (the Chair of the Senate Human Services Committee). These distinguished women then spoke to parents and professionals at a women's forum that we sponsored about the needs of individuals with FAS and their families. At that time they all made personal commitments to develop public policy that works for those individuals disabled by prenatal alcohol exposure.

The FAS Advisory Panel

Mary Lowry became dedicated to FAS issues. Due to her influence, Governor Mike Lowry appointed a Governor's FAS Advisory Panel in the fall of 1994. Mary Lowry graciously consented to serve as the honorary chair over the panel. It was the responsibility of this panel to compose a report on FAS, complete with recommendations for the future direction of Washington State public policy, practice and procedure regarding FAS. A healthy percentage of parents were appointed to the panel including three members of the FAS Family Resource Institute. The report and recommendations were completed and presented to the Governor in January, 1996.

Legislation on FAS

In the Spring of 1995, SSB 5688 was signed into law. The first section of this law appropriated funding for the development of tools to diagnose disabilities caused by prenatal alcohol exposure, and to provide training for diagnostic teams around the state through the University of Washington. Dr. Sterling Clarren has led this pioneering effort to ensure that individuals disabled by prenatal alcohol exposure have timely access to an accurate diagnosis. Vicky McKinney, the current co-director of the FAS Family Institute, was invited to serve as the parent advocate trainer on the FAS Clinical Network Team.

The other opportunity mandated by this law was an FAS Interagency Agreement. As directed by the law:

> "The Department of Social and Health Services, the Department of Health, the Department of Corrections, and the Office of the Superintendent of Public Instruction shall execute an interagency agreement to ensure the coordination of identification, prevention, and intervention programs for children who have fetal alcohol exposure, and for women who are at high risk of having children with fetal alcohol exposure. The interagency agreement shall provide a process for community advocacy groups to participate in the review and development of identification, prevention, and intervention programs administered or contracted for by the agencies executing this agreement."

The resultant agreement, finalized before the end of 1995, states that in addition to the above mentioned agencies, the signers of this agreement, including the University of Washington, the FAS Family Resource Institute, and the March of Dimes, agree to the following:

> *Vision: To prevent alcohol-related birth defects and to make it possible for affected individuals to achieve their full potential through client/family centered services.*

> *Beliefs: FAS/FAE diminishes the quality of life for effected individuals, their families, and communities; FAS/FAE results in significant social, legal, economic, education, and health problems; FAS/FAE is totally preventable; early identification and intervention offer the greatest hope for reducing the negative consequences of FAS/FAE.*

The group that assembled to draft this document was excited about the possibility of continuing to serve the state in overseeing the implementation of the agreement. Thus the FAS Interagency Work Group (IAG) was born. Ann Waller and I serve on this committee with the responsibility of representing family FAS advocates across the state. We believe that this window of opportunity has extensive and immense possibilities for changing public policy and practice in Washington State.

In June 1996, Governor Mike Lowry appropriated money from the state emergency fund to continue a prevention project that had proven successful: Dr. Ann Streissguth's Birth to 3 Project. This project, which was in danger of being discontinued for lack of funding, supports mothers who are at risk for giving birth to children with FAS and who are attempting recovery. Governor Lowry had by this time come to recognize the critical need to prevent future births of children with FAS, to the extent that he was willing to field criticism for using emergency funds. We commend Governor Lowry for his courage in supporting this and other FAS prevention projects.

In addition to these successful events, one other major product of our efforts, in collaboration with other advocacy groups, was Washington State Liquor Control Board's requirement to display FAS prevention signs at all points of alcohol purchases in Washington State.

Funding for the FAS Family Resource Institute

At the heart of all our advocacy activities was our desire to protect, provide and care for our own children. This passion goes beyond money, career advancement, embarrassment and credentials. For four years, we operated without outside funding. Our endeavors were accomplished through donated time, resources and cooperation and collaboration with other disability and mental health advocacy groups, other parents and professionals. Although this put a severe strain on our family budgets, this allowed us to be free from contractual obligations which might have limited or altered our activities. In 1993, we made a difficult decision to reject an offer of full funding because that offer would have tied us to the mission and agenda of another organization that was not focused on the needs of individuals disabled by prenatal exposure and their families. Finally, in 1995, Ken Stark, the Director of the Washington State Division of Alcohol and Substance Abuse (in the Department of Social and Health Services), officially contracted with us to fund three very important products: our quarterly newsletter, a toll-free crisis and information phone line, and statewide trainings for parents and professionals.

As our families fell into the traumatic conditions which prompted personal action, embers of hope generated desperate searches to save our families. We discovered answers in the form of help and support from other parents and professionals. We were able to create opportunities and use them as catalysts for change. We generated events and products that served as change points that moved us further toward our goals. When we reflect on the results of our efforts and advocacy, we face the future with confidence that public policy and practice in Washington State will continue to transform into one that works for individuals with FAS and their families.

Spider Web Walking:
Hope for Children with FAS Through Understanding

Jan Lutke

A few months before I was asked to write this chapter, a remarkable thing happened. My daughter, who was 12 at the time, had been asked to speak to a group of teachers about what it was like to have FAS. She asked me if she could practice what she wanted to say, using me as her audience. She proceeded to draw for me and explain the wonderfully apt analogy that is the basis for this chapter. She uses this analogy to explain FAS, and she calls it "spider web walking." She drew a picture of a very lopsided spider web of big holes and broken strands. This web represented her brain. She explained to me that having FAS was "like having a broken spider web in my brain. Sometimes I get to stick just right and I can do it, and sometimes I fall through the holes and I can't." I was amazed at her perception and questioned her further. I asked her if the reason she "fell" was because she could not do the task at hand. She very carefully explained that I had misunderstood her. The reason she could not do the task was precisely because she fell. In other words, the fall came first. I sat mesmerized as she told me how she had to "walk" on the spider web and how difficult that was. She had just summed up accurately, in a few minutes, what had taken me years of concentrated thought and effort to learn! All this from a child who is still unable to do multiplication tables, cannot tell time, and does not know left from right. Miracles do happen, if we but take the time to hear them.

I remember very clearly the day, more than ten years ago, when I began the process of understanding what "spider web walking" meant for the affected individual. I happened to be flipping though a dictionary, looking up the word "accessory." In one of those minor detours from a task we all take, memorable only for the inconsequential nature of the event, my eyes were drawn to the word "abstract." I read the definition, which I remember as "a thought apart from any particular object or real thing, but somehow related to it — *a lump of sugar is real; the idea of sweetness is abstract.*" I was intrigued by this definition. I sensed that I was on the edge of something important to my understanding of how children with FAS seemed to act, but I was not sure just what it was.

At the time, I had over 10 (now over 20) year's experience in dealing with the behavioral and emotional challenges related to issues of abuse and neglect in adopted and foster children; in fact, dealing with these issues had become a way of life for me. I gradually was incorporating into my normally good parenting skills an aware- ness that children with FAS were different — in how they approached just about everything — from other behaviorally and emotionally challenged foster children. I had parented children diagnosed with FAS for over five years. I had read everything I could about FAS, gone to workshops, liaised with medical professionals and other parents, and was in the beginning stages of setting up a support network. It was a "teachable moment" for me — I was open to hearing and seeing things differently.

Experience over the years has taught me the value of moving slowly. I decided to let this thought on the elusive nature of abstrac- tion sit and percolate for awhile. Over the next few months, I spent a lot of time thinking about this idea. Children with FAS have great difficulty with abstraction and conceptual thinking, and I thought about the relationship of the nature of abstraction to the interven- tion strategies that I used. I knew that these strategies worked, but I came to understand that I really did not know why they worked, except in the most cursory way. They were "successful accidents."

It occurred to me that I should give equal consideration to the "concept" piece of the equation. What are concepts anyway? Where do they come from? Why do we have them? Concepts are ideas which are formed and understood in the mind — this seems obvious. What may be less obvious is that the mind is the only place a concept exists. Even more obscure is the process of conceptualiza- tion.

We often try to work in the middle of a problem, instead of figur- ing out where its beginning is, and I wanted to get to the beginning of the problem of understanding children with FAS. I was struck by the obvious but still elusive applicability of these definitions to what we see with FAS. What intrigued me was the idea that these defini- tions were important to understanding the specific problems children with FAS seem to have, especially social and behavioral problems.

The end result of this personal learning process that I just have described has been the development of an operational paradigm for understanding and intervening with FAS based on these fundamental components of "spider web walking." Understanding and using conceptual thinking, understanding cause and effect, generalizing information, understanding time, and utilizing short-term memory. To deal effectively with life itself, to be able to function, one must be able to use these processes on a very sophisticated level of accomplishment. We take these processes for granted. If people with FAS are unable — not unwilling — to do this on our terms, in our ways, is it possible that they could use external processes to replace those internal ones which they do not have?

Problems with Understanding and Using Conceptual Thinking

Abstractions and concepts work together to simplify and put order into what would otherwise be a world of overwhelming complexity. Concepts provide guidelines and parameters for our functioning, and usually are taught parent to child, generation to generation. Social values for human interaction are concept-based. Accurately understanding and using concepts permits an individual to understand what is required of him/her in a particular situation and to predict how he/she will need to act in future similar situations. Using concepts allows one to predict the how, what, where, and when of an interaction. I understand that the concept of "one" can be 24 (one day) or 7 (one week) or 30 (one month) or 365 (one year), depending on which concept of "one" I am using at that moment. I understand the concept of the word "if" and when to apply that idea. I understand that a moving car is real, and that the concept of danger associated with that car is also real, even though I cannot see, hear, or feel that danger. There are many different variables which determine the level of danger in any given instance, including what I do. I am lucky. My brain *automatically* sorts through what it knows about a particular situation and, unless I am very unlucky, comes up with the right choice for action. For the person with FAS, this critical process of understanding and applying concepts and abstractions to particular situations is neither automatic nor consistent. "Spider web walking" becomes difficult and fraught with pitfalls.

Problems with Memory

People with FAS often have difficulty with storage, integration, or retrieval of information, and this difficulty has a negative impact on one's ability to adequately and accurately address a situation requiring a response. For people with FAS, information sometimes is stored in a random, haphazard fashion, with no predictable order. Even when information is stored in the right file cabinet under the right file code and in the right file, it tends to "get lost." It seems to disappear without warning, only to reappear, unpredictably, right where it should be. These unpredictable memory lapses and gains happen just often enough to convince those who do not understand FAS that they are deliberate "behaviors" under the control of the person with FAS. The reality is very different. No one is more frustrated by this situation than is the affected person, who must continually deal with the reactions of other people. Telling the truth, making sense of situations, and responding to requests become difficult. Even when information has been successfully stored and accessed the individual with FAS must be able to interpret what he or she needs to do with that information. "Lying" is a by-product of these difficulties. It occurs when interpretation of what was originally stored incorrectly runs headlong into a distorted perception of the environment and one's relationship to it.

Understanding Cause and Effect, Generalizing, and Problem Solving

For people with FAS, an understanding of the relationships between cause and effect can be missing altogether, available only sporadically (when you stick on the spider web), faulty, or just not an automatic process. Linking causes with effects, and remembering these links, allows one to generalize information from one situation to another. The ability to generalize information is a basic prerequisite for problem solving. It allows one to be flexible and to check out possibilities and shift them around — an important middle step in any problem solving process. Looking at all the pertinent factors which apply to a situation allows one to come up with the appropriate action for a situation. If you do not have the ability to think about different possibilities, your ability to make good choices based on possible outcomes will be altered.

People with FAS often do not have all the pieces of the puzzle, and if you change one piece of the puzzle you may have a completely different puzzle. A situation may appear to be entirely new, and any previous learning, even if retained, does not seem to be relevant. Everything that happens is unprecedented; past experiences and social rules are not linked to situations. All too often in FAS, the first choice is seen as the only choice, even when the solution clearly does not work. When someone with FAS appears to show no remorse for an action, it may simply be because the "possibilities" piece of the equation is not there.

Problems with Motivation

Reflection, something most people do in a split second, is a very complicated function. It comprises many inter-related thought processes, any one of which, if faulty, will radically alter the way in which one perceives relationships between people, things, or events. Reflection is control. Motivation is a problem when this function is missing, especially when there are no immediate or concrete outcomes for a behavior. Without the ability to reflect, to consider possibilities, to imagine outcomes, there is no reason for effort. Would you be motivated to make changes to things if you were unable to understand and keep the connections between the potential changes and your actions?

Problems with Time

Time is an anchor which places humans in relationship to others and their environment: We know where we are and who we are. Our anchor does not move. It allows us to swing in a circle — a cycle — and when one cycle is completed, we start over again, or incorporate the first cycle into a bigger one. Always, the anchor holds us in place, giving us crucial stability. With FAS, this anchor finds no secure hold, and the line of time simply unravels endlessly with no clear beginning and no clear end. People with FAS are frequently oblivious to our form of time. They do not show up for work on time, come back late from coffee, miss appointments, forget to eat, do not know what day of the week it is, and seem unable to complete a task even when they know the steps. Nothing gets done the way it is supposed to get done. Time does not pass, it simply *is*. Combine a poorly secured anchor with difficulty sequencing and with difficulty grasping the floating concept of "one" as it relates to time, (whether one hour, one class, one coffee break or one rinse cycle) and you may have great difficulty functioning. "Telling time" on a clock becomes a major frustration. It demands the generalization of concepts from math, the use of "before and after" concepts, approximation, an understanding of similarities and differences, knowing up from down and right from left, and the ability to hold *all* of this in your head at the same time, and not get distracted in the process. You must remember what you did not understand to start with and recognize the need to do the same thing all over again at some future point which remains unrecognized. Then, of course, you need to connect the numbers on the clock to the task at hand which is a different process altogether!

Most people possess an internal time clock that allows them to "sense" time, which is compatible with the natural order of things and into which concepts can be incorporated. People with FAS do not possess this clock.

Missing Connections — the Spider Web Theory

The concurrent use of memory, cause and effect, generalization and time skills allows us to make logical, rational and sensible decisions about what should be done, when it should be done, and who should do it. FAS critically impacts one's ability to make sense of the environment, to communicate effectively, and to problem solve. Once the fall-out from problems requiring abstract thinking and memory are understood, it becomes very clear that people with FAS will have great difficulty in making sense of the world, even in the absence of problems with attention and activity. In fact, those children with FAS with good memory, higher IQ and without obvious attention problems seem to have even more problems, probably because our expectations are affected by what we see as fewer disabilities related to prenatal alcohol exposure. It has been my experience, however, that losing the edge on abstract thinking is all it takes to produce very significant functional deficits. Connectors are missing, and connections are what are crucial.

Consider how physical connectors work. A kitchen tap with a defective washer will spray water in all directions instead of in a steady stream; an electric kettle with an unseen break in the cord will boil water some of the time and not others; if the cord linking the VCR to the TV is not screwed in tightly, the picture will be fuzzy — three different connection problems, each of which causes the job to be incompletely or inconsistently done. How difficult would it be to wash your hands if the water was spraying all over? You have the soap, the scrub brush and the towel, but still your hands are not clean. The connector to bring the water in touch with your hands and the soap at the same time is not working. Transfer this idea to a mental process and you begin to have a sense of what is actually going on with people with FAS. You know the "what" and the "how" but you do not know the "when" and the "why." The "spider web" has broken, or perhaps the strand was never there.

Our job is twofold: Strengthen the "spider web" if we can, and catch the falling spider when we cannot.

Re-Weaving a Stronger Spider Web

What are the properties of a spider web? It is a resistant, flexible but fragile structure, firmly anchored on at least four points. A spider always builds a web the same way, using a series of connecting strands. The structure serves the spider well. If something breaks the connecting strands, the spider falls on a silken parachute which protects it from harm.

The FAS spider web has an oversized weave so that information falls through. Sometimes the strands are weak and break easily. Other times the web is too sticky and information cannot pass along it. Frequently, the web does not connect where it is supposed to connect; it lacks order.

Like a spider web, our thought processes are intricately connected. If the strands randomly break, could we not, like the spider, reconnect them? We need some sort of support mechanism that can strengthen the strand sufficiently for a connection to occur. Could we build new strands across some of the holes in the web to spread the spider's weight over a bigger area? Could we loosen the perseverant glue when we need to? In fact, successful "accidental strategies" work precisely because they strengthen the spider web!

Understanding the spider web gives us the most crucial piece of this puzzle. We must realize that *at the heart of all compliance issues is a competency issue.* We have to move from seeing behavior as *noncompliance* to seeing it as *non-competence*. This critical perceptual shift allows one to stop "doing to" and start "doing with." It permits the art of spider web walking.

I experienced the most enormous relief when this change took place. Suddenly, I knew I was okay and so were my children. I began to hear them differently, to experience them differently, and finally, to understand them differently. I recognized if they could not adapt to the complex, complicated and constantly changing world, then I would have to be the one to adapt, because I am the one who is able to do so. Now I envision the environment as the spider web, our attitudes, advocacy, home and school as the anchor points, and supervision as the parachute.

Being part of a spider web is a difficult task. There are so many places where the web can break. I have learned to take responsibility for only those things over which I have control. The choice of reaction or response to a situation is mine. If I simply react, neither the child nor I learn very much; we simply experience another frustration. If I take the time to respond, which requires viewing a behavior or a problem in light of what I know about abstraction, I may be able to repair or strengthen the spider web. Responses take more time than reactions. Responding requires that I become a student of behavior, always asking what the underlying concept involved might be, and how I could potentially take what is abstract and make it concrete. It is a constant challenge, and there are as many setbacks as successes. How I view these setbacks makes the difference. Reweaving a spider web is a work in progress. One must not lose sight of the fact that the spider must continue to operate while the work goes on. If, in our desire to reweave, we fail to secure the anchor points or pack the parachute, we risk harming the web walker.

Reweaving the web itself can be done in as many different ways as there are ideas. *The key is to work smarter, not harder.* Reduce the need to generalize and comprehension is significantly improved. Use every sense to teach and connections are improved. Conceive of time as a straight line instead of a circle and its passage can be taught. Use symbol language, color and music to fill in the holes and memory can be triggered. Develop routines which allow a child to "know" where he or she is. Fill in the blanks and relationships between things may become easier to grasp.

Although we cannot repair the spider web once and for all, we can strengthen it sufficiently to allow at least some improved functioning. Improved functioning leads to improved self-esteem, an important protective factor. Good self-esteem leads to a willingness to try.

Children and young adults with FAS are remarkably resilient people. If we can make the shift to incorporate the way they learn into the way we teach, we open up new possibilities for success.

A few years ago, a national "think tank" conference on FAS was held in Canada. My oldest daughter with FAS, who was 17 at the time, was asked to speak to the assembled delegates at the luncheon. She had attended the morning session and listened to a Federal Government Minister talking about the "victims" of prenatal alcohol exposure, and commenting repeatedly on all the things they could not do. Although she had not comprehended much of the speech, what she had understood bothered her. She fumed through the rest of the morning and I was a little concerned about a "rescue plan." However, I need not have worried. In fact, I have never been as proud of her as I was during her presentation. What she told the delegates at the end of her talk is the essence of the paradigm shift that all of us who live and work with FAS know to be true, "There are two things I want you to know: Do not call me a victim, and do not tell me what I can not do. Help me to find a way to do it."

If we can keep these two things in the forefront of our thoughts, we will have moved from doing "to" to doing "with" for people with FAS.

We will have joined them on the spider web.

Residential Programs for Persons With FAS: Programming and Economics

Joseph J. Hess, Jr. and George W. Niemann

Introduction

Fetal Alcohol Syndrome (FAS) is the primary cause of mental retardation in the United States (Abel & Sokol, 1987) and leads to the placement of thousands of children and adults in various health and human service facilities. However, due to the particular characteristics of FAS (Steinhausen, Nestler, & Spohr 1982; Dyer, Alberts, & Niemann, 1995), many victims remain undiagnosed and, without adequate early intervention, develop secondary disabilities that often result in placement in juvenile justice and other inappropriate systems (Streissguth, Barr, Kogan, & Bookstein, 1996).

Providing effective treatment programs for individuals with FAS requires the development of environments conducive to positive treatment outcomes. This chapter will discuss both the programmatic and economic pros and cons associated with congregate (i.e., institutional) and community-based models of residential programs and advocate for the development of a continuum of services for individuals with FAS.

Programming

The field of developmental disabilities has led healthcare and human services in developing models of service delivery which seek to provide treatment in least restrictive settings. Over the past twenty-five years large state-run and private institutions have been replaced with an extensive array of community-based alternatives for the delivery of services. The range of options includes group homes serving ten or more individuals to supervised apartments serving one or two.

In considering the development of residential programs to address the needs of persons with FAS, it is important first to understand the impact which community-based models of delivery have had elsewhere in the field of developmental disabilities. Fortunately, some important longitudinal studies have identified some key programmatic considerations.

The Pennhurst Study

The Pennhurst Longitudinal Study detailed the effects of deinstitutionalization (Conroy, 1995). This study followed 1,154 people who formerly lived at the Pennhurst facility in Pennsylvania and were transferred into community living arrangements starting in 1978. The population included individuals who were nonverbal (50%), suffered seizures (33%), were at least partially incontinent (47%), demonstrated aggressive behaviors (40%), and were labeled severely or profoundly retarded (85%). The individuals studied moved from a large institutional environment to three-person living arrangements in the community with day services provided outside of the living environment. Annual surveys and interviews with these individuals and their families have been conducted over the past eighteen years, and will continue to be conducted in the future.

Regarding quality of life, the Pennhurst study found that, after moving from an institutional to a community-based setting,

- 14% of the clients improved their self-care skills;
- Challenging behaviors lessened by an average of 6%;
- Health remained stable and use of medications dropped slightly;
- Life satisfaction ratings doubled; and,
- Participation in structured day programs increased from 33% to almost 100%.

Regarding the impact of deinstitutionalization on the community,

- Over 90% of the families of people with disabilities noted satisfaction at some level with the community program;
- 75% of the neighbors of individuals living in community living arrangements were unaware of the existence of the program; of the 25% aware of the program half were positive about the program. Indications were that neighbors became positive as the program continued over time; and,
- The average per diem cost of care was nearly 15% lower in the community than in the institution.

The Pennhurst study suggests that community-based programs are potentially more programmatically effective than are their institution-based counterparts.

Bancroft's Studies

At Bancroft, a 114-year-old private organization serving over 850 individuals in southern New Jersey and mid-coast Maine, a comprehensive program evaluation system has been installed to measure the quality of life of individuals served. This system allows for analysis of the effects of Bancroft's many components. Bancroft's studies suggest that a community context — one that encompasses a number of options permitting individuals to progress toward maximal independence — meets the goals of individuals served more effectively than does a community context that does not encompass different options (Hess & Niemann, 1995). In general, the data from Bancroft's studies supports the finding that a continuum of community-based services is necessary to achieve maximal independence for individuals served.

As Bancroft developed a comprehensive continuum of services in the community it became obvious that some individuals, during periods of decompensation and regression, would require periodic, short-term intensive intervention that could not be delivered safely and effectively in the community. Individuals with FAS also will occasionally experience acute episodes of behavioral crisis (Dyer, Alberts, & Niemann, 1995), requiring intensive support and treatment for some period of time in order for them to regain independence and continue to maintain themselves in a community setting. Without some form of safety net, individuals who experienced acute crisis while living in community-based environments had no alternative other than psychiatric hospitalization. Generally, it was Bancroft's experience that these individuals rarely returned to their former level of independence — if they returned to Bancroft at all —after such hospitalization. In Bancroft's experience, providers cannot afford to depend on psychiatric institutions to adequately address the unique needs of individuals during such acute episodes.

In response to this problem, Bancroft designed a unique neuro-behavioral stabilization unit on its main campus in Haddonfield that could handle individuals during acute episodes of behavioral or medical crisis. The organization built three single-family-styled homes on the campus. Each home was designed to serve up to five individuals in private bedrooms with all of the amenities of a family home. Each unit contained hidden monitoring and security systems. Windows were made of unbreakable lexan and alarmed. Ceiling heights were raised by one foot and air exchange was increased dramatically to enhance freshness and comfort. A special dry-wall material called "Fiberbond" was imported from Canada and installed throughout the units for safety and maintenance purposes. Extensive landscaping helped hide stockade fencing used to secure individuals from elopement.

The program, dubbed the "Lindens," provides intensive behavioral evaluation, treatment planning, intervention as well as step-down and maintenance levels of service designed to effectively transition persons back to the community in a minimal period of time. The program provides an alternative to psychiatric institutionalization for persons who otherwise can live more independently in the community. As such, the Lindens fills what had been a void in the Bancroft community-based continuum of services, permitting individuals to "tune up" when necessary without risking the loss of gains they previously worked so hard to achieve.

Since its inception in 1995, the Lindens program has currently served 53 individuals in severe behavioral crisis, effectively returning 92% of them to community settings in an average of 53 days. While the cost of providing such services averages over $750 per day per client, the program is far cheaper than comparable institutional settings charging close to $1,500 per day. Moreover, individuals are transitioned back to their community settings with behavioral plans and specific prescriptions for staff to follow in reintegrating these persons back into a normal life style. This component of Bancroft's continuum of services is vital to the success of our community-based programs and recommended for other providers looking to establish an effective network of community-based services for persons with FAS.

Programming Conclusions

Some conclusions can be drawn from both formal deinstitutionalization studies and Bancroft's experiences in the delivery of community-based services that might help guide the development of residential programs for persons with FAS:

- There is no single community-based alternative to institutional care. A continuum of services is necessary to address the needs of individuals with disabilities such as FAS.

- A comprehensive continuum of services provides an intensive back-up support for persons in periodic acute crisis.

- A comprehensive continuum of services provides a variety of community-based programs that foster independence over the life cycle of individuals needing service.

Individuals with FAS require structured settings to be able to function effectively (Dyer, Alberts, & Niemann, 1995). Without the appropriate structure, individuals with FAS may develop "secondary" disabilities (Streissguth, Barr, Kogan, & Bookstein, 1996) and tend to spiral downwards and get into trouble with the law. It is imperative, therefore, that they be provided with highly individualized settings to meet their unique needs for structure. A continuum of services ranging from the intensive to the less intensive offers such individuals a broad range of options for structured living and learning. Structure can be varied on a continuum to tailor programs to meet the unique needs of each individual with FAS and allow him/her to experiment with greater levels of independence.

Economics

As noted in the findings of the Pennhurst study, the average cost of community-based services for the individuals studied was approximately 15% lower than was the cost of institutional placement. Unfortunately, this statistic might lead to unintended conclusions that could affect public policy and result in a disservice to individuals with disabilities, including individuals with FAS. To understand the situation completely, the economics of community-based delivery models must be understood.

One of the key economic considerations in the care of individuals with developmental disabilities, including FAS, is that individuals who require residential placement very likely will require such support for the duration of their lives. Given that the average life expectancy of persons with developmental disabilities is now catching up with the average life expectancy of the population as a whole, the "length of stay" that might be expected of individuals in residential placement eclipses fifty or more years. With this in mind, the measure of the cost effectiveness of services is longitudinal in nature, with peaks and valleys occurring at various times over the life span.

Clearly, given these economic realities, an individual's achievement of programmatic goals will influence the overall cost effectiveness of service delivery. As individuals become more independent, costs should decline, with periodic requirements for additional support during occasional crises being the exception rather than the rule. A community-based continuum of services can handle this situation nicely.

There are important differences between community-based and institutional settings with regard to staffing, facilities, food services and transportation. These differences should be taken into consideration when addressing the residential needs of individuals with FAS, particularly if a provider's experience is largely institutional (i.e., residential treatment facilities and other similar settings).

Staffing

Staffing community-based programs presents a far different challenge than does staffing institutional settings. Figure 1 compares the full-time equivalent (FTE) staff requirements of institutional settings to those of community-based programs, using Bancroft's data. As indicated, for individuals with moderate to high intensive requirements, staff costs are going to be *higher* in community-based settings than in institutional settings.

Generally, this cost difference is driven by the environments in which these programs take place. For example, in an environment such as a group home for five individuals, the ratio of staff to persons served has a limit of one-to-five. However, in an institutional setting, the ratio might be one-to-ten or larger and still enable the institutional caregiver to provide "line-of-sight supervision" to all individuals on the unit. In Bancroft's experience, this situation changes at minimum supervision levels, when individuals are able to live independently in the community with direct staff supervision of only several hours per week.

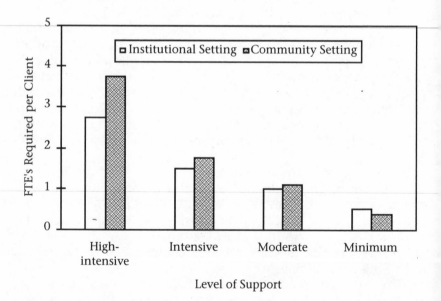

Figure 1. Number of full-time equivalent (FTE) staff in institutional and community settings.

Some of the increase in staffing costs for community-based programs will be offset, however, by a decrease in expenditures on *facilities*. Figure 2 compares facility expenditures per client in institutional settings to community settings. As indicated, facility related costs are *lower* in community-based settings. However, several factors peculiar to Bancroft's system impact this cost difference. First, by policy Bancroft does not utilize group homes for more than five individuals, in order to avoid the development of a "mini-institution" in the community. Second, Bancroft almost exclusively utilizes leased properties. This allows Bancroft to avoid major front-end capital expenditures, transfers the risk of maintaining major systems like heating, ventilation and air conditioning to a third party, and retains operating flexibility in the event that a relocation is necessary.

Another cost which is lower for community environments is *food*. Providing centralized commissaries is a costly ordeal; there are staff costs for central food purchasing, food preparation and clean-up. Significant capital expenditures are necessary for the provision and maintenance of central food services. Figure 3 compares the costs of salaries/benefits and food/supply purchases of institutional and community-based settings. Since food preparation and clean-up activities are vital components of community programs, staff direct

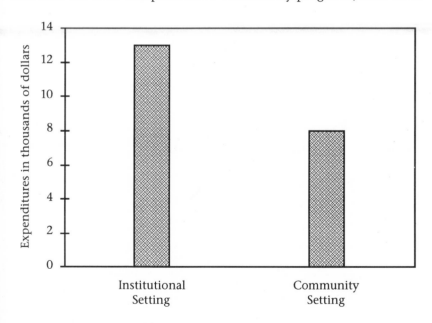

Figure 2. Facilities expenditures per client in institutional and community settings.

residents in these areas, thus avoiding the cost of separate food preparation staff. Buying food and supplies from local markets is a more expensive proposition than group purchasing, but programmatic gains for individuals served far outweigh this minor cost difference.

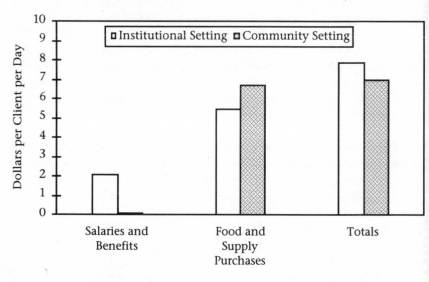

Figure 3. Food costs.

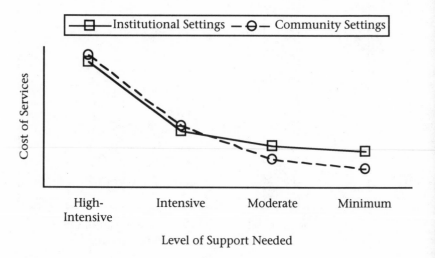

Figure 4. Relative overall cost of services.

Transportation

Costs are far higher in the community than are transportation costs in more self-contained institutional or campus settings. This cost is further increased if the community residence is not close to an effective public transportation system. Licensing requirements mandating a vehicle in the community for each location of five or more people is a factor in New Jersey.

Economic Conclusions

When all is said and done, the average cost per day to serve an individual in the community rather than in an institutional setting will depend on the level of independence achieved by the client group as a whole (Figure 4). A comprehensive community-based continuum of services can address this situation by providing individuals with a progression of steps toward greater and greater independence, thus reducing the total cost of care over time.

A continuum of services, when spread out through a large community, requires an effective system of staff training and support. Staff Development and Program Evaluation are important cost factors that cannot be underestimated in the provision of community-based services, particularly for individuals with FAS. In Bancroft's experience, this investment in the training and proficiency of staff adds approximately $1,187 per annum to the cost of caring for an individual. However, there are few investments which pay off as handsomely for the individuals served and the organization as a whole.

Public Health Implications of FAS

Richard J. Jackson

The potential for fetal exposure to alcohol is huge. Here are some facts:

- Among women, all forms of drinking, including the most harmful forms (heavy drinking and binge drinking), are most common among those in their twenties — the age range when childbearing peaks. Approximately 40% of women in their twenties report drinking to the point of intoxication within the preceding 12 months (Wilsnack, Wilsnack, & Hiller-Sturnhofel, 1994).

- About half of pregnancies are unintended, and up to one in ten women may not recognize their pregnancy until the second trimester. Thus, a fetus may be inadvertently exposed to alcohol during its early development (Forrest, 1994).

- Among women who delivered infants in 1988, about one in five reported alcohol consumption around the time of conception, about one in twenty reported drinking after recognition of their pregnancies, and about one in two hundred reported heavy drinking during pregnancy (Journal of the American Medical Association [JAMA], 1995).

As someone who is not an expert on Fetal Alcohol Syndrome (FAS), I am impressed by the parallels between FAS and other public health problems that are more familiar to me. For example, there are lessons to be learned from the public health realms of lead toxicity prevention and smoking cessation. In this chapter, I will briefly review the progress made in preventing these other public health problems, and suggest applications of these prevention lessons to the prevention of fetal exposure to maternal alcohol.

Progress in Prevention of Lead Toxicity

In 1980, the most widespread toxic exposure affecting children in America was lead. Each year, more than 200 million pounds of lead were dispersed into the environment through the tail-pipes of American automobiles. Half of the older homes in the United States had lead-containing paint. Infants consumed lead in milk because cans of formula were contaminated or because maternal milk was contaminated by the lead in mother's bodies. The consequences of in-utero lead exposure are not unlike those of alcohol exposure. Lead damages developing brains. Fetal exposure to lead is associated with impaired ability to socialize and may contribute to delinquency later in life.

Just as there were multiple sources of lead contamination, there were multiple approaches to solving the problem; and there was competition among those who thought they had the best approach to preventing lead exposure. Experts in housing, water, and air pollution competed for scarce public resources. While advocates for prevention of lead poisoning competed among themselves, there were powerful industries — automotive, gasoline, paint, and the lead industry itself — that were committed to maintaining the use of lead in a variety of products. In fact, the lead industry once claimed that lead was an essential ingredient in the human diet. We now know that there is no safe dose of lead.

As with fetal alcohol exposure, lead exposure was common; lead use was promulgated by large and powerful industries; there were multiple and competing approaches to addressing the lead problem; and exposure to lead had widespread and lasting effects on the health and development of children.

But there has been dramatic success in the lead poisoning prevention story. Over the past two decades, expectations about achievable levels of exposure have changed and the prevalence of elevated blood lead levels in the population has declined. When I was a medical student, nearly half of the children on a pediatric ward during one of my rotations in New York City were hospitalized for treatment of lead poisoning. At that time, the working definition of lead poisoning was a level greater than 60 micrograms per deciliter (µg/dl). By the time I was in residency training, the definition of lead poisoning was a level greater than 40 µg/dl. By the time I began my career in public health, it was down to a level greater than 20 µg/dl. Now it is a level greater than 10 µg/dl. When I was in training, few people imagined that average blood lead levels in children could ever be reduced to less than three µg/dl. In the 1970s, average blood lead levels in children were in the range of 13-14 µg/dl, a range now considered toxic. In 1990, six years ago, the average blood lead level in children younger than five years of age was 3.8 µg/dl, approaching what was once thought to be the irreducible minimum.

We have had tremendous success in removing the toxicant lead "from upstream in the pipe line." It is difficult to prevent or control contaminants at the milligram level. It is much easier to prevent exposures when you are talking about box cars and tank cars and pipelines. Tons of lead were removed from gasoline, and tons of lead were removed from paint. If you go back to that same hospital in New York now, you do not see wards full of children receiving treatment for lead poisoning. This is because we have lowered the level of lead in American children. Because the overall levels of lead are so much lower, the number of children with toxic exposures also is dramatically lower.

Progress in Smoking Cessation

Another pervasive and harmful exposure to the developing fetus is cigarette smoke. It is helpful to reflect on the dramatic changes that have occurred in social attitudes toward smoking. There was a time when medical journals in this country carried advertisements depicting physicians smoking and touting the health benefits of smoking. Changing these attitudes has required that powerful industries be challenged, industries that continue to wield enormous power in Washington D.C., in state legislatures, and at certain times in local boards of supervisors. Who would have imagined five or ten years ago that the President of the United States would announce at the White House that this country is going to reduce smoking and that the focus of these efforts would be the protection of children and young adults?

At the very minimum, if we can get young people to postpone experimenting with tobacco, we will reduce the number of kids who become addicted. Any delay in the onset of an addiction is to the good. Any reduction in the total number of cigarettes that someone smokes in a lifetime is to the good.

The social environment is also very important. We are concerned not only about the health of smokers but about the health of those whose exposure to tobacco smoke is passive. The public pressure that has led to the prohibition of smoking in an increasing number of public buildings has arisen largely from concerns about environmental tobacco smoke. "We do not want your toxic habit affecting our health," say nonsmokers.

Lessons from Lead Toxicity and Smoking Prevention

One lesson we can learn from the prevention of lead poisoning and addiction to tobacco is that it is important to take a long-term view. We must not allow ourselves to be too discouraged when short-term progress is modest. There are reasons for our modest progress. Although cultural beliefs that exposure of the fetus to alcohol is harmful date to biblical times, prevailing social attitudes towards drinking have led to an acceptance of drinking during pregnancy. This behavior continues to be widespread.

Another lesson we can learn is that work with individuals and families affected by fetal alcohol exposure must be complemented by public health policy approaches aimed at preventing fetal alcohol exposure. The recent report on Fetal Alcohol Syndrome by the Institute of Medicine (Stratton, Howe, & Battaglia, 1996) emphasized several priority areas that require development, including two areas that are important components of a public health approach to the prevention of fetal alcohol exposure: improving our understanding of the epidemiology of FAS and developing interventions to prevent alcohol-related fetal damage.

To shape public policy, one must have data. How many people are affected by this problem? What is its impact? If you do not have documentation, policy makers are not swayed. Estimates of the extent of FAS and associated morbidity vary considerably, reflecting variations in levels of alcohol consumption in different populations as well as variations in data collection methods. At the Centers for Disease Control and Prevention (CDC), we have been working to improve methods for public health monitoring of FAS through collaboration with selected state and local health departments.

We also must have information about "what works." Where should the government put its money? What efforts should be supported? At the CDC, we have been supporting selected state and local health department programs to develop prevention efforts among women at highest risk of delivering alcohol-affected children. CDC also proudly supports the work of Dr. Streissguth and her colleagues. The body of information they have collected is a milestone in documenting the impact of Fetal Alcohol Effects on children and in guiding approaches to preventing secondary complications.

Having answers to these questions also is important in changing policies of large managed care organizations. Our ability to convince managed care organizations to address fetal alcohol problems will depend on our ability to demonstrate that these are important problems and that feasible interventions will have an impact on these problems. We can have a voice in helping to shape the public's expectations about what constitutes quality preventive care in these organizations and in shaping the "report cards" that society is demanding of these health care providers.

The Alcohol Pipeline

Like lead and tobacco, there is a "pipeline of prevention" for alcohol. For alcohol, that pipeline is fueled by a massive advertising effort, and much of that advertising reaches children and teens, offsetting our efforts to relay messages about the hazards of alcohol exposure during pregnancy. For example, during the 1996 Summer Olympic Games held in Atlanta, advertising promoting alcohol use was pervasive at the Games themselves, on television, and in sports magazines. We know that prohibition — a strategy that attempted to completely close down the alcohol pipeline — did not work, but we must confront the powerful messages delivered to our children and seek to delay and lessen alcohol use. Compare the sophisticated advertising that promotes alcohol with the modest warning by the Surgeon General on alcohol containers. This warning may have as its greatest impact the exemption of manufacturers from liability.

So how should we think about slowing the flow of the alcohol pipeline to young people and pregnant women? Just as there were those worried about housing, paint, water, and air pollution around the issue of lead poisoning, there is an array of groups worried about alcohol's impact on our children. There is tremendous diversity when you consider all those who share our concerns about fetal alcohol exposure. This diversity could be a hindrance or a source of strength. Certainly, many who have been affected by this problem have an historical reason to distrust those of us who represent government agencies. Yet, in an environment of scarce public resources, we must collaborate. We must continue the dialogue about these issues that has begun and seek ways to focus our collective strengths. With our diversity and collective strength we have tremendous power to impact this problem.

Rapporteur's Report:
A Summary of the Conference

Fred Bookstein

The international conference that inspired this book, "Overcoming and Preventing Secondary Disabilities in Fetal Alcohol Syndrome and Fetal Alcohol Effects" was held on September 4-6, 1996 at the University of Washington Health Sciences/Medical Center, in Seattle, Washington. This conference was sponsored by the Fetal Alcohol & Drug Unit of the University of Washington's School of Medicine (Department of Psychiatry and Behavioral Sciences) and the Disabilities Prevention Program of the Centers for Disease Control and Prevention (CDC).

The conference gathered together people from around the world to discuss the problem of secondary disabilities in people prenatally affected by alcohol. Although over 60 speakers presented information and ideas at this conference, only a few of these presentations could be transformed into the chapters that comprise this book. This chapter briefly summarizes most of the remaining presentations. It is hoped that the interested reader will get a small taste of some of the other material presented at this conference, and will become acquainted with some the many excellent researchers, professionals, parents and other advocates who are working hard to push our field forward and tackle the problem of secondary disabilities.

Session 2: New Studies on FAS/FAE

A Longitudinal Study on FAS from Germany
Hermann Löser, M.D., College of Medicine, Wilhelms University, Germany

Germany has the highest national average of ethanol intake per capita, about 12 liters per year. More than one percent of our newborn deliveries are to alcoholic mothers. In 1975, we therefore determined to carry out a study of children of chronic alcoholic mothers. Forty-two percent of the sample were FAE, and 13% were the most severe (Type III) FAS. Fifty-two of the 336 subjects are now adults. Of these 52, only half are expected to function independently; the rest need sheltered surroundings. All newborns began around the third population centile in size, height, weight, and head circumference. Height and weight now tend to be in about the 20th centile, except for a subset of females who have become quite fat, although head circumstance for these women remains at the third centile. Forty-one percent of these subjects last attended a regular school — but none attended gymnasium (college-preparatory school), although 39% of the normal population attends gymnasium. Tests of thought disorders showed delayed, viscous thinking, inflexible, without fantasy. Their behaviors showed persistent infantility and unrealistic play. There was not much aggressiveness, trouble with the law, or sex offenses. Vocationally, none of these adults were professionals, and more than half were in the simpler occupations. I conclude from all this that the permanent part of the damage due to alcohol is much worse than we thought. FAS/FAE is not a personality type, rather, a pattern of malformations. It is best to place these children in supportive foster families. Of the interventions appropriate for secondary disabilities, I believe the most important is to prevent alcoholism among people with FAS; this should not be too difficult once they are identified.

Neuropsychological Deficits in Memory
Kris Kaemingk, Ph.D., Department of Psychology, University of Arizona

We compared 20 children with FAS/FAE, aged 6 to 16 years, to age-sex-matched normals. Three kinds of memory were tested: verbal memory (story memory, sentence memory, and sequence memory), visual memory (a copy task, a change detection task), and learning (verbal and nonverbal recall). The children with FAS/FAE differed from the others in all three areas and on most of the individual tests. These findings are consistent with the general belief that children with FAS "live in a new world every day." Still, they have a learning curve — they benefit from repetition. I recommend that we decrease the load on their memories by use of memory aids, by management of parental demands, and by reliance on strict routines for activities such as hygiene that can be carried out in exactly the same sequence every day. Children with FAS/FAE are best taught one-on-one, with no distractions.

Identifying Deficits in Social Communication
Truman Coggins, Ph.D., Department of Speech and Hearing Sciences, University of Washington

Speech pathologists have tests for everything, but most of these tests have no social validity. What parents report about children with FAS indicates that *social communication* is their most pressing problem. They are talkative but not communicative — loquacious but typically off the mark. They have poor judgment and social skills, lack social savvy, and cannot understand the motives of others. Our clinic assesses narrative productions. We evaluate the coherence and cohesion of connected discourse — its informative and logical properties — and the use of language to regulate social interactions or thinking. Children who lack these skills are at great academic risk. We also assess mental state reasoning, that is, the knowledge of other minds. Children with FAS are very weak in both these areas.

Session 3: Mental Health and FAS

Mental Health and Family Issues
Marceil Ten Eyck, M.C., C.C.D.C., Psychotherapist, Washington, and Diane Malbin, M.S.W., FAS Counselor and Consultant, Oregon

Marceil Ten Eyck: It is not only people with FAS who have secondary disabilities; so have their families. Absent a proper diagnosis, when you devote all that love and effort to parenting and it's still not OK, counselors tend to blame us parents — "if only you'd been a better parent . . ." — but, worse, we tend to blame ourselves. It is crazy-making to be told that there is nothing wrong with your child under these circumstances. The child's behavior is attributable to real brain damage. Once this is discovered, there is a real grief process. If the community or the state continues to deny the diagnosis, then is the time for rage. Everyone involved in these tragedies is in profound pain. Burn-out benefits nobody; take care of yourselves and the rest of your family as much as you take care of your child with FAS.

Diane Malbin: Diagnosis actually can do the child with FAS a great deal of good. It is not that I *am* the problem, but that I *have* a problem. After all, children with FAS, like the rest of us, have the need to make sense of their own behavior. In the absence of a diagnosis, well-meant interventions and therapies can be horribly inappropriate. Children with FAS force us into a major paradigm shift in our professions, a merger of brain function with behavior. We must acknowledge, for instance, that learning theory is about most, not all, brains. FAS children tend to violate the axioms of most established learning theories, and so the interventions they impute rarely fit the needs of children with FAS. The fact of the diagnosis itself, of course, is just such a paradigm shift, at the level of the individual child; it must precede all the others.

An FAS Study on a Child Inpatient Psychiatric Unit

Karen Kopera-Frye, Ph.D., Department of Psychology, University of Akron

Beyond the general population of people with FAS, one ought not to ignore the special populations in institutions such as hospital wards or prisons. In this study, 330 consecutive admissions to a children's inpatient psychiatric facility were studied to document alcohol exposure and its relation to dysmorphology referral and, ultimately, to behavior problems. Our data arose solely from review of charts — we encountered only paper, not patients. Of the cases we reviewed (mostly white males), 269 of the 330 charts indicated that a question about maternal alcohol use had been asked — this is good news indeed. There were 57 mentions of alcoholism associated with gestational use, and 37 referrals to dysmorphology. Of the 23 children seen by a dysmorphologist, 8 were diagnosed FAS and another 8 as variants of FAE. The rate of fetal alcohol diagnoses on this ward is manyfold higher than is the general population base rate of 1 to 3 per thousand live births.

FAS and County Mental Health

Charles Huffine, M.D., King County Division of Mental Health, Washington

Treating FAS/FAE children requires clinicians to consider differential diagnosis. One must assess functional disabilities and understand the developmental impact of those disabilities. Moderately impaired individuals can be treated in an office practice setting. More severely impaired individuals will need an array of services from such systems of care as Division of Developmental Disabilities, Department of Child and Family Services, Division of Juvenile Rehabilitation, and Mental Health. Currently our systems of care are often fragmented. King County, Washington, is exploring models of integrating care. A grant project is considering the possibility of blending funds from various systems for the most disturbed children and coordinating all services under one care manager. This model is based on high involvement of families in plans for particular children as monitors of the blended funding program.

FAS and Psychopathology

William Sherman, M.D., Eastern State Hospital, Washington

As our inpatient institutions continue to empty, more and more people with FAS/FAE turn up in community mental health centers. These are old-timers, often profoundly retarded. At the institutions, they all have been put on Mellaril, a psychotropic drug that dampens behavior sometimes to the point of catatonia. How do you diagnose these people without medical records or parents? One way is to slowly reduce the dose of Mellaril and see what symptoms first emerge. Often one finds what Clarren called "the atypical FAS profile," accompanied by post-traumatic stress syndrome because of all the abuse suffered in the institution. These people have high risk of serious depression and of temporal lobe seizures from being hit on the head. They often have behavioral repetitions and stereotypies, and turn floridly psychotic under stress. In Spokane, we are establishing a teaching clinic for these and other developmental disabilities out in the community. It is going to be the primary care physician's task to carry this load; but at present we do not know what advice to give this physician.

FAS, Attention Deficits, and Medications
Alan Unis, M.D., Department of Psychiatry, University of Washington School of Medicine

Wender's Law of minimal brain dysfunction states that anybody can respond to any drug at any time. FAS is of high clinical complexity, with a phenotype only now being defined. We have little wisdom to offer about psychotropic medications, in particular to parents who have learned a justifiable suspicion of the mental health system. Just as there is no "typical" psychopathology of the FAS case — some come in hyperactive, others oppositional — the client's response to medications is likewise unpredictable, with a high rate of adverse side effects. Be careful!

Session 4: FAS and the Schools

What the Child with FAS Needs from School
Ann Waller, M.Ed., FAS Family Resources Institute, Washington

Raising a child with FAS is a team project, in which the schools must do their part. A student with FAS needs trained staff (from administrators to teachers to nurses to bus drivers) who understand this disability. This student also needs parents knowledgeable in advocacy techniques, Individual Educational Plans (IEPs), an appeal process, and, throughout all of this, interdisciplinary staffing. These information and planning meetings may be set up through a referral or "focus of concern." These meetings are necessary so the child's needs can be addressed from all perspectives, including the parents'. The student needs Special Education eligibility under the category of "health impaired." This can help the student by establishing eligibility regardless of IQ level or academic performance, and by documenting disability for other situations, such as SSI (federal disability) eligibility or trouble with the law. Finally, the student needs DDD (state Department of Developmental Disability) eligibility and School to Work Transition Program eligibility. An IEP is mandated to have transition goals and objectives by the time the student is 16 years old. This transition should prepare and assist the student's move into appropriate supported employment.

Special Education for FAS/FAE in Juvenile Corrections
Mary Ann Rothwell, M.A., N.C.S.P., Echo Glen School, Washington

Echo Glen is a juvenile correction facility in the Washington woods, off Interstate 90, for 220 young inmates, half of whom are violent offenders. Many of the males are sex offenders as well. Many of these youth were prenatally exposed to alcohol; many have problems of drug and alcohol dependency themselves. Nationwide, 45% of incarcerated offenders are eligible for special education. Our task was to make this place less like a junior high school — to give these kids life/social/job skills — in the face of the inevitable need for security. There is a lot of behavior control, of course, and time on task is "paid." The emphasis throughout is on learning by doing. Fractions are taught by cooking, for instance, and adding and subtracting are taught by using the student store. There is a flower shop and a greenhouse in which these educationally disadvantaged youth (don't you dare call them "delinquents") actually grow things. We have a speech and language pathologist who educates the *staff*, and many, many surrogate parents. What works is clear: base teaching in lifelike activities, structure, repeat, simplify, individualize. But why did these kids have to get locked up to be successfully schooled? — why can't we contribute resources to their education at an earlier age?

Developing a Teacher Training Model for FAS
Charles Schad, Ph.D., Department of Education, Black Hills State University, South Dakota

In 1991, the South Dakota school system totally lacked any knowledge of FAS. Superintendents had never heard of it, teachers were not helped to cope with it, and their professors never talked about it. One day, though, some of us visited Seattle and Fairbanks and discovered that we had the same problem as these other places. Our main task became to train teachers in detection of the possibility of FAS and in the response once it is diagnosed. The main goal of training should be to pick up every *new* entry into the professions. We have decided to put in place a certification requirement, and a module in undergraduate and graduate curricula of education. The overall process took about two years in this rural state, but it is now in place.

Session 5: Employment and Independent Living

When the Child with FAS Grows Up
Wilma Robinson, R.N.B.S., Mental Health Coordinator, Ute Mountain Ute Tribe

My own adopted child was born with FAE along with many other anomalies, such as a club foot. As a child, he had frequent ear infections and many other difficulties. His IQ exceeded 100, but the Performance IQ/Verbal IQ differential was 28 points, a fact we did not learn until he was in junior high school. He failed in college, could not gain certification from a vocational training program, and now works as groundskeeper for a golf course. He has the classic FAE temperament, with no recognition of boundaries. He cannot manage delayed gratification; he has the normal obsessions and concerns of anyone of his emotional age, which is about 15. Quite engaging, he nevertheless was not able to hold his marriage together. My son cannot ever manage money, totally misses all social cues, and is completely incapable of abstract thinking.

Getting Along in Life: A Basic Skills Training Program
Sandy McAuliff, M.S.W., Adolescent Clinic, University of Washington School of Medicine

Although we do not currently have an FAS clinical treatment protocol, I think it is important to look at effective protocols addressing related problems like ADHD and Borderline Personality Disorder. We could begin using these interventions and adapting and customizing when necessary in order to develop an FAS protocol.

The diagnostic category of Borderline Personality Disorder (BPD) sounds a lot like the FAS stereotype: impulsiveness, affect instability, lack of planning skills, and outbursts of anger. For people like this, Marsha Linehan's Dialectical Behavior Therapy (DBT) Skills Manual for Borderline Personality Disorder may prove effective. The goal of DBT is to teach emotional regulation, and to avoid the high reactivity and slow return to baseline that seems to characterize these people. Part of BPD results from an invalidating environment in which communication of private experience is met inappropriately or frankly pathologized. In DBT, one is taught not to drive the therapist crazy. The targets of DBT are mindfulness, distress tolerance, and regulation of inner response. These targets often are achieved in individual cases.

Session 6: FAS and Sexuality

FAS Adolescent Sexuality Through the Eyes of Parents
Linda LaFever and Vicky McKinney, FAS Family Resource Institute,
Washington

Danny is 14 years old, five foot four, 110 pounds, very innocent, very naïve, and in acute late stage testosterone poisoning. Alas, sexuality is one of the aspects of behavior that FAS does *not* diminish. Because of his naïveté, my son, who was the March of Dimes' first FAS poster child, has had two serious molestations in his life, one quite recently. Thirteen-year-old Abby McKinney is mentally retarded, so her parents can outwit her most of the time — and yet it is necessary to think toward a future of sexual activity. Older FAS girls seem accepting of Norplant, but it does not protect against sexually transmitted diseases. The thought of sterilization is abhorrent — yet I know I personally would pay most of the price of any unwanted pregnancy of Abby's. This daughter of mine, who is a healthy person with FAS, is "betrothed" to Danny, even though he has been heard to declare, "She is too FAS for me." You *must* take the scientific findings about secondary disabilities into your communities, and say: If you do not do these things, then my child has no future.

Sexuality in People with Disabilities
Steve Sloan, Ph.D., Sex Therapist, Georgia

It's the able-bodied who have problems with sex and sexuality. In populations like people with FAS, so very vulnerable, these issues must be confronted long before the problems arise, which is to say, long before the typical parent is comfortable talking about them. At every age there are appropriate issues that can be raised usefully. This requires some compromise of the child's innocence, but, after all, guilt and shame do not reduce the extent of sexual behavior: They merely increase our obsession with it. The best protection against abuse is high self-esteem, a training which begins earliest of all. Remember, too, that abstinence is never a cause of death, and even married people do not have to bear children; this can all be taught to the very young.

One suitable topic of discussion is masturbation. What an irony that Jocelyn Elders was fired for discussing it! — it is the most riskless of all sexual behaviors. Young men with FAS do not seem to have lower testosterone levels; what are they supposed to do about it? Masturbation is, for instance, far less likely to become a problem than is acting-out of sexual impulses. People with FAS, like any other innocent or disabled people, have sexual impulses, but also the ability to control them.

A particular aspect of the FAS phenotype that affects sexuality, I imagine, is the ADHD part, with the concordant need for immediate gratification; the distractibility component, though, can also lead to sexual dysfunction. We are quite familiar with behavior modification techniques that can control this disability. (We typically do this better for females than for males.) Like other aspects of sex education, this need not be IQ-dependent. One can role-play how to say "No" or teach the limits of appropriate touching. Depression, which seems high in some people with FAS, is a complicating factor here. It does not reliably decrease sexual desire—indeed, adolescents often indulge in sex as a "quick fix"—and antidepressant drugs often have sexual side effects, such as paraphilias.

In many disabilities, including spina bifida, the main protection against inappropriate sexual behaviors is social skills. For persons with FAS, too, it is essential to practice how to reliably read interpersonal cues. We need to prepare the mentally handicapped for situations in which they will be abused. They need to learn what is inappropriate touching by others, and when to scream. That 82% of the mentally handicapped are sexually abused is obviously a social problem, not a psychiatric one.

Session 7: Criminal Justice and FAS

Identifying and Serving Youth with FAS in Detention
Julianne Conry, Diane Fast, and Christine Loock, University of British Columbia

The following information represents our preliminary findings from a one-year study that is nearing completion. We have studied 44 youth with a history of prenatal alcohol exposure who were inpatients in the provincial youth forensic facility for British Columbia and the Yukon. While there is increased awareness of FAS in our legal circles, the ordinary procedures of rehabilitation do not seem to alter problem behaviors. By screening this population, we are attempting to detect youth with FAS and FAE as a first step toward more humane alternatives. Ultimately, our job is to assist physicians, psychologists, lawyers, judges, and teachers to better understand and serve these youth. The level of social competence in these youth can be typified by this quote from a staff person: "Every time he gets sent to his room, he needs a complete explanation."

British Columbia has about 300,000 youth aged 12 to 18; on a typical day, about 300 are in custody. Our Inpatient Assessment Unit houses ten at a time, totaling about 300 per year. In our study, all youth were given a thorough physical and neuropsychological assessment. We also measured the usual facial stigmata of FAS and obtained a history of prenatal alcohol exposure. To date, out of the 215 screened, 44 appear to be afflicted to some extent. Of these, three met the diagnostic criteria for the full FAS according to IOM criteria, the rest being FAE (partial FAS or ARND). The total prevalence of alcohol-induced deficits is thus about 20% of this population. Of the 44, 80% were male; 44% white. Their median IQ was 89. The most diagnostic physical feature was short palpebral fissure length. Youth came from a variety of living situations, mainly foster or group homes. A significant number never lived with their birth mother; none lived with both parents. More than half of them had been abused physically, emotionally, or sexually, and more than half had a prior history of trouble with the law. Eighty percent had attention deficits, 56% had a history of substance abuse, and 30% had a conduct disorder. Half were labeled "learning disabled" and there was typically a pattern of disrupted schooling.

Behaviorally, these youth were characterized as demanding, loud, lacking modesty or awareness of personal boundaries, socially inept, concrete in their thinking, with high need for acceptance, moody, and disinhibited about the discussion of personal information. This matches the classic behavioral profile of people with FAS/FAE that is emerging from the Seattle research group.

We conclude that there are disproportionately many youth with FAS/FAE in the inpatient psychiatric assessment unit of the juvenile justice system of British Columbia and that screening for these conditions is feasible. Our work increased staff awareness of this type of young offender. Judges, lawyers, psychologists and psychiatrists are now considering the possibility of these diagnoses. Still, many people with FAS/FAE do not pass through this system. Hence, early diagnosis is critical, as is life in a stable living situation with compassionate caregivers.

Impact of an FAS Identification Study on Washington State Prisons
Robert Jones, Ph.D., Chief of Clinical Services, Washington State Department of Corrections

When I was first introduced to FAS it became clear that in Corrections we had been working with offenders suffering from this problem for years. However, we were not aware of the dynamics of these problems or how they should be addressed. When Ann Streissguth came to us with her proposal for a detection study, we took it as an opportunity to sensitize the staff to this class of offenders. The experiment worked: Treatment policies have been changed, staff have increased their interest in programs, and offenders are being addressed according to their unique needs. In the Washington State system, intake procedures have been altered to incorporate a history of alcohol exposure. It has taken an enormous load off of the corrections staff to be able to understand why offenders behave the way they do rather than simply attribute it to "antisocial" behavior.

A Criminal Justice Experience
Barbara Wybrecht, R.N., Parents Supporting Parents, Michigan

I thought my son had escaped most of the pain of the person with FAS. He was a higher-functioning case, diagnosed as an infant the very first year the diagnosis became available. Up until age 21, with his entire family serving as advocates, he was coping well: no discipline problems, no lying or stealing, no school disruptions, no employment problems. Unbelievable. And yet, at age 21, his world came crashing down. He was interrogated by the police without an advocate present. Unable to sense danger, he sees everybody as a friend. This trusting 9-year-old in a 21-year-old body simply could not understand that he *must not* talk to police. There needs to be some sort of card summoning an attorney for every person who, like my son, is cognitively challenged. My son, under interrogation, confessed to the alleged crime.

We reached out for assistance. We will never know the truth of the case, probably. Two consultants decided that no crime had occurred. Do we try to educate a judge, or a jury? On advice, we pleaded "no contest" and tried to affect the sentencing. To our horror, we failed: Our son was sentenced to two to fifteen years. This was terrifying, given our son's desire to please and his inability to tell safety from danger. We knew that in custody the lessons he had learned with such difficulty at home would be lost, the man returned to us far less functional. Fortunately, he felt safe, even in prison. Mom and Dad called every day, and a familiar therapist visited him regularly. We solicited postcards for him from all over the country, and an enormous network of support finally resulted in a resentencing: home on probation. (The prosecution is appealing.)

In my son's case, clearly, it took a village to raise a child with FAS, a national "village." Likewise, it will take whole villages to overcome the other secondary disabilities of FAS, and, ultimately, to prevent them.

Session 8: Native Americans: Special Issues and Programs

Introduction
Philip May, Ph.D., Department of Sociology and Psychiatry, University of New Mexico

I want to correct a misconception regarding the incidence of alcoholism in Native American communities. More so than many other communities, most Native American tribes have many more abstainers than problem drinkers. Moreover, their communities have traditional values about alcohol as strict as they are about most other concerns. There is, however, a problem subset of binge drinkers. This is not due to any biological difference in alcohol metabolism or alcohol dehydrogenase deficiency (although of course there are individual differences) — the problem is sociocultural.

Most importantly, we need to acknowledge the contributions of Native American sharing, experience and data to knowledge of FAS. The effect of increasing maternal age was first noted in studies of Native Americans; likewise the problems of the multiple-FAS family, and the association between FAS and premature maternal death. Also, Native Americans are responsible for some of the best case management schemes we have. In general, keep in mind that culture affects not only the secondary disabilities of FAS/FAE, but also the primary problem and the corresponding primary, secondary, and tertiary prevention strategies.

Indian Health Service Programs on FAS
Eva Smith, Ph.D., and Marlene Echo Hawk, Ph.D., Department of Alcoholism and Substance Abuse, Indian Health Service Headquarters West

The Indian Health Service is changing dramatically as a result of federal downsizing and the shifting of resources directly to tribes. This includes the loss of three Headquarters West staff and several full-time Area Coordinator positions. Many of the patient education and resource materials are now available from the National Clearinghouse on Alcohol and Drug Information rather than from our office.

The program is community-based and multi-disciplinary in its approach to public health. All providers, physicians, nurses, psychologists and social workers must share in prevention, intervention and case management, but also must work closely with families and local community structures. Primary prevention targets not only risk factors for substance abuse but also the strengths that exist within the family, local community and culture. There is a strong wellness and sobriety movement among American Indian/Alaska Native (AI/AN) communities. Indian Health Service plays a small role in supporting this grassroots effort through the funding of prevention and treatment programs.

A recent evaluation of AI/AN women's treatment services (the majority of which are run by tribes and native organizations) found that women wanted to be good mothers and that that was often a motivating factor for women seeking treatment services. Comprehensive alcoholism and substance abuse treatment for women *is* FAS prevention.

The findings from the studies presented at this conference show that early diagnosis and intervention make a difference and will assist our ongoing efforts to train providers to diagnose and get past the attitude of not wanting to "label" a child. Our office has plans to develop training materials for behavioral health providers on treatment strategies as well as materials for parents and caregivers.

An important element to always remember that is basic in native communities, but applies to other cultures as well, is that everyone has a spirit and addressing that spirit should be considered in prevention, intervention and treatment work.

Traditional Approaches to FAS Healing
Carolyn Hartness, FAS Educator, King County Department of Public Health and Eastern Band Cherokee Nation

I speak on behalf of Rick Two Dogs, a Lakota healer from South Dakota, who was unable to be present here because of illness in his family. I will share Rick's and another Nation's healers' successes using ritual to dramatically alter the lives of people with FAS.

There is a particular strength of Native American cultures that can serve as a crucial part of caregiving for people with FAS. Traditionally, those who are "different" are more closely connected to the realm of the Spirit. They are to be respected for that reason alone. Many of the behaviors of people with FAS that are labeled "secondary disabilities" correspond to traditional roles in Native American communities, such as the one who hears voices. People with FAS thus have many good qualities, and, if raised in a context of unceasing support for their self-esteem, become as integral to their communities as can any other member. To that end, please remember that language is powerful. These are not "FAS kids" but "children with FAS," and their mothers are not "alcoholics" but "women with alcoholism."

Session 9: Public Health, Screening Tools, and Diagnostic/Service Programs

New Screening Tools for the FAS Face

Susan Astley, Ph.D., Departments of Epidemiology and Pediatrics, University of Washington School of Medicine

A unitary score for "FASness" of a face, like grams of birthweight or points of IQ, will increase diagnostic accuracy and open many doors that children and families with FAS need opened. This paragraph summarizes a full report that recently appeared in the Journal of Pediatrics. Of eleven measures of 27 children considered to have the classic facial phenotype of FAS, three indexes were found to be consistently anomalous: palpebral fissure length, smooth philtrum, and thin upper lip. We devised objective formulas capturing some of the information available to the diagnostician from each of these features. In a discriminant analysis of 42 FAS cases against 42 controls, validated using another 42 controls, it proved possible to classify the 42 FAS cases unerringly by a formula combining the ratio of palpebral fissure length to inner canthal length, the ratio of the area of the upper lip to its squared perimeter, and the clinician's judgment of smoothness of philtrum on a 1-to-5 scale. Our formula can be expected to aid in clinical case definition, in screening, and in rehabilitation.

The Fetal Alcohol Behavior Scale

Helen Barr, M.A., M.S., Fetal Alcohol & Drug Unit, University of Washington School of Medicine, and Fred Bookstein, Ph.D., Institute of Gerontology, University of Michigan

We developed a scale sensitive to the behaviors (not the facial characteristics) typical of the person with FAS/FAE. It applies across age, sex, ethnicity, and IQ and seems quite promising for both detection and screening. We began with Ann Streissguth's clinical checklist of odd behaviors that her clients' mothers often mentioned, and after analysis ended up with a sublist of 36 behaviors. The reliability of this scale, the Fetal Alcohol Behavior Scale (FABS), is very good, about .90. The median score in our clinical population is 21, versus around 7 in a normal comparison group. The score turns out to be almost perfectly *un*correlated with age, IQ, sex, or diagnosis (FAS or FAE), so that no adjustments are required. In a prison population, of the four cases highest on this score, three reported exposure to alcohol and also had low IQ or a history of seizures, two bits of evidence for the CNS damage we are searching for. In a population of ordinary children seen at a family clinic in Seattle, the FABS score was associated with maternal drinking history but not with paternal drinking history. In our large study of secondary disabilities, a low FABS score seems nearly essential for success at employment and for independent living. We recommend use of this checklist as a screening tool for FAE in clients aged two and above whenever there is known prenatal exposure or known CNS damage. The correlation of this and other neurobehavioral measures with brain damage as measured neuroradiologically is an area of active research at this time.

An FAS Diagnostic and Service Center for High-Risk Mothers and Babies

Maria Ferris, M.D., K.I.N.D.E.R. Clinic, University of Texas–Houston Medical School

The K.I.N.D.E.R. (Kids In Need of Drug Evaluation and Rehabilitation) Clinic is Houston's only comprehensive long-term program for substance-exposed infants. The families are disorganized, of course, and access to health care is invariably burdensome. Over the years, we have come to solve this problem by a systematic expansion of the clientele from the child himself/herself to other exposed children and then to the family unit. We operate a comprehensive primary health clinic for these families, including some of the ancillary services they so obviously need. Main funding is from the Texas Department of Health, with the help of Hermann Children's Hospital and the University of Texas–Houston Health Science Center. Among our most useful innovations has been the creation of a "passport" that accompanies our clients when they need to visit emergency rooms, a small document listing crucial facts relevant to their emergency care.

We are also active in the matter of restaurant signage about drinking during pregnancy. At present our efforts entail the voluntary posting of our signs (which imitate Washington's) across the restaurants of the Houston area. We are doing well in this effort.

Session 10: Responses to FAS by Institutions and Families

Organizing for FAS at the National Level: The March of Dimes, The Arc, and NOFAS

Richard Johnston, M.D., Medical Director, March of Dimes, Washington, D.C., Kathy McGinley, Ph.D., Assistant Director, Office of Governmental Affairs, The Arc, Washington, D.C., and Todd Donaldson, Assistant Director, National Organization on Fetal Alcohol Syndrome, Washington, D.C.

Richard Johnston: I am not an expert on FAS, but I have a deep concern for the problem. The March of Dimes (MOD) has the potential to participate with you in addressing the problem of FAS, and I urge everyone to make a tie-in with their local MOD. MOD is a grass-roots organization with local chapters in every state. Each chapter has a Health Professional Advisory Committee and it is here that people can infiltrate the MOD and become members. The committee conducts needs assessments and develops program plans for education, advocacy and services. MOD's mission is to improve the health of babies by preventing birth defects and infant mortality. We focus on pre-pregnancy care, prenatal care and care of newborns and infants. Our overall strategies include research (molecular as well as clinical), advocacy (state and congressional) regarding public policy, education, and provision of community services. MOD distributes pamphlets and videos on alcohol and pregnancy and has developed a substance abuse curriculum for obstetrics residents. I was appalled when I heard Michael Dorris talk of obstetricians who recommended martinis to pregnant women; maybe our curriculum will help eliminate such advice. Through our MOD Resource Center you can get information on referrals to other organizations, community services, national advocacy, etc., all accessible via e-mail as well as the Internet.

Kathy McGinley: I have passion and interest, but not expertise on FAS. I am an advocate in D.C., where I would be called a lobbyist, but because I lobby for good things I consider myself an advocate. The Arc is the largest national organization devoted to voicing the needs of people with mental retardation and their families. Because FAS is the leading preventable cause of mental retardation, prevention of FAS is one of our major goals. We have taken a multi-dimensional approach with activities in the areas of education and outreach, legislation, research and action on a national, state and local level. We look at everything that has an impact on the life of a person with a disability, including housing, money, education, and civil rights. We are active in expanding FAS prevention programs; our focus on specific legislation addresses the dangers of alcohol through warnings on radio and TV alcohol advertising. We were successful in getting warning labels on alcoholic beverages. We introduce FAS legislation every year; with Representative Joe Kennedy we have been a voice against the alcohol industry's use of the airwaves to glamorize drinking. Our 1200 local chapters are very active in disseminating materials on FAS, education and outreach work and legislative advocacy. We need grassroots efforts in this work.

Todd Donaldson: The National Organization on Fetal Alcohol Syndrome (NOFAS) is a non-profit organization focusing totally on FAS. We rely on foundation grants, and corporate and individual contributions to conduct our efforts. Patti Munter founded NOFAS in 1990 after having worked on reservations in New Mexico and South Dakota where she met many children with FAS. She went back to Washington D.C. where she started a newsletter and set up a national information clearinghouse to bring national resources together. We have a number of programs, one of which is to develop other model programs that can be replicated. The first such program was a medical school curriculum for first and second year medical students that we pioneered in 1992 in New Mexico; this has now been replicated in several other places. We also spend our efforts collaborating with various educational and health organizations to distribute information on FAS. We have worked with the NEA to distribute 100,000 copies of an FAS Handbook and recently we have worked with state HMO coordinators to provide information on FAS. In D.C. we are working with teens to teach them about alcohol and its effects.

Organizing for FAS at the State Level
Kenneth Stark, M.B.A., Director, Division of Alcohol and Substance Abuse, Washington State Department of Social and Health Services

The task of a coordinator, whether at the state or local level, is to coordinate people, not systems. Coordination is communication. Here in Washington, with the legislature's explicit blessing, we have put together an interagency work group on informational and collaborative projects on FAS. The group includes staff working on identification, prevention, and intervention, and people interested in advocacy, research, and administration. It is essential to bring together groups this diverse if the available funds are to be spent effectively. Another group, the Washington Interagency Network, deals with issues of alcohol and substance abuse more generally. They, too, agree to keep talking, to fund joint activities, and the like.

Groups like these are easily influenced by advocates. Advocates have more leverage, in fact, than most academic researchers or other experts, because advocates have the passion and the stories that sway so effectively. Local groups of parents or other providers can network into these groups. If you, all of you, push at the same time on the same specific agenda, you will change public policy: There is no doubt of this. The key to dealing with government, at any level, is mustering collective pressure toward sufficiently specific initiatives.

Organizing for FAS at the Local Level: The Family Empowerment Network, and the March of Dimes
Moira Chamberlain, Coordinator, Family Empowerment Network, University of Wisconsin, and Nancy White, Past Director, Programs and Communication, Western Washington March of Dimes

Moira Chamberlain: The Wisconsin Family Empowerment Network serves the needs of Wisconsin families with FAS. It distributes resource lists, matches parents to local service providers, runs an annual retreat for families that includes child care, organizes teleconferences, arranges for home visits and publishes a newsletter.

Nancy White: The Western Washington March of Dimes emphasizes the three C's: communication, collaboration, and chocolate. Communication — get volunteers involved, know their strengths, ask for what you need. But, also, acknowledge our *own* need to help, and do not patronize. Instead, remove the moral asymmetry. Collaboration — our best effort ever is the Fabulous FAS Quiz Show video, now distributed widely by the Department of Schools. Keep your door open for unexpected pro bono efforts, like the freelance poster designer who dropped in a while ago. Track down resources used by women of childbearing age, like the commercially available "preconception calendar," and add messages about alcohol to them. Do not be afraid to take your expertise right to the Rotunda of the State Capitol; we were integral to the passage of the bill funding the Diagnostic and Prevention Network of Washington State. Finally, the Internet is free. FAS web sites are popping up all over the place; *use them.* Chocolate — one of the pleasures of service arises when you remember to honor each other. The pleasure of chocolate reminds one, also, that service to the FAS community is a daily matter. Hopelessness and anger cannot sustain community support; the advocate is partly responsible for insuring that the community understands all the issues day by day.

The conference ended with Robin LaDue's videotape, "Tribute to Children." As the faces of child after child with FAS came before us, the murmur of the old hymn "Amazing Grace" passed from the soundtrack until all of us filled the hall with it. May it continue to resonate far beyond the confines of these three conference days, until people with FAS are all treated with humane understanding even as we prevent others from being born as they were.

References

Aase, J. M., Jones, K. L., & Clarren, S. K. (1995). Do we need the term "FAE"? *Journal of Pediatrics, 95* (3), 428-430.

Abel, E. L. (1990). *Fetal Alcohol Syndrome*. Oradell, NJ: Medical Economics Books.

Abel, E. L., & Sokol, R. J. (1986). Fetal alcohol syndrome is now the leading cause of mental retardation. *Lancet II,* 1222.

Abel, E. L., & Sokol, R. J. (1987). Incidence of Fetal Alcohol Syndrome and economic impact of FAS-related anomalies. *Drug and Alcohol Dependence, 19*, 51-70.

Abikoff, H., & Gittelman, R. (1985). The normalizing effects of methylphenidate on the classroom behavior of ADHD children. *Journal of Abnormal and Child Psychology, 13,* 33-44.

Abkarian, G. G. (1992). Communication effects of prenatal alcohol exposure. *Journal of Communication Disorders, 25,* 221-240.

Alin-Åkerman, B., & Nordberg, L. (1980).Griffiths' utvecklingsskalor I och II. *Manual for Administering och utvärdering*. Psykologiförlaget Stockholm.

Aman, M. G., Marks, R. E., Turbott, S. H., Wilsher, C. P., & Merry, M. B. (1991). Methylphenidate and thiordazine in the treatment of intellectually subaverage children: Effects on cognitive-motor performance. *Journal of the American Academy of Adolescent Psychiatry, 30,* 816-824.

Amaro, A., & Hardy-Fanta, C. (1995). Gender relations in addiction and recovery. *Journal of Psychoactive Drugs, 27*, 325-337.

Aronson, M. (1984). *Children of alcoholic mothers.* Unpublished master's thesis. University of Göteborg, Göteborg, Sweden.

Aronson, M., Kyllerman, M., Sabel, K. G., Sandin, B., & Olegård, R. (1985). Children of alcoholic mothers: Development, perceptual and behavioral characteristics as compared to matched controls. *Acta Paediatrica Scandinavica, 74*, 24-35

Aronson, M., & Olegård, R. (1987). Children of alcoholic mothers. *Pediatrician, 14,* 57-61

Astley, S. J., & Clarren, S. K. (1995). A Fetal Alcohol Syndrome screening tool. *Alcoholism: Clinical and Experimental Research, 19,* 1565-1571.

Autti-Rämö, I., & Granström, M. L. (1991). The psychomotor development during the first year of life of infants exposed to intrauterine alcohol of various duration. *Neuropediatrics, 22,* 59-64.

Barkley, R. A., McMurray, M. B., Edelbrock, C. S., & Robbins, K. (1990). Side effects of methylphenidate in children with attention deficit hyperactivity disorder: A systemic, placebo controlled evaluation. *Pediatrics, 86*, 184-192.

Barnard, K. E., Magyary, D., Sumner, G., Booth, C. L., Mitchell, S. K., & Spieker, S. (1988). Prevention of parenting alterations for women with low social support. *Psychiatry, 51*, 248-253.

Barr, H. M., Streissguth, A. P., Darby, B. L., & Sampson, P. D. (1990). Prenatal exposure to alcohol, caffeine, tobacco, and aspirin: Effects on fine and gross motor performance in 4 year old children. *Developmental Psychology, 26*, 339-348.

Beery, K. E. (1989). *Manual for the developmental test of visual-motor integration*. Cleveland: Modern Curriculum Press.

Bierich, J. R., Majewski, F., & Michaelis, R. (1975). Fetal alcohol syndrome. *Pediatric Research, 9*, 864.

Bihrle, A. M., Bellugi, U., Delis, D., & Marks, S. (1989). Seeing either the forest or the trees: Dissociation in visuospatial processing. *Brain and Cognition, 11*, 37-49.

Bowman, J. (1994). *Washington state needs assessment survey on Fetal Alcohol Syndrome effects*. Seattle, WA: James Bowman Associates.

Brown, R. T., Coles, C. D., Smith, I. E., Platzman, K. A., Silverstein, J., Erickson, S., & Falek, A. (1991). Effects of prenatal alcohol exposure at school age. II. Attention and behavior. *Neurotoxicology and Teratology, 13*, 369-376.

Burd, L., & Martsolf, J. T. (1989). Fetal alcohol syndrome: Diagnosis and syndromal variability. *Physiology & Behavior, 46*(1), 39-43.

Chandler, L. S., Richardson, G. A., Gallagher, J. D., & Day, N. L. (1996). Prenatal exposure to alcohol and marijuana: Effects on motor development of preschool children. *Alcoholism: Clinical and Experimental Research, 20*, 455-461.

Chernoff, G. F. (1977). The Fetal Alcohol Syndrome in mice: An animal model. *Teratology, 15*(3), 223-229.

Clarren, S. K. (1977). Central nervous system malformations in two offspring of alcoholic women. *Birth Defects, 13*, 151-153.

Clarren, S. K. (1986). Neuropathology in Fetal Alcohol Syndrome. In J. R. West (Ed.), *Alcohol and brain development*. New York: Oxford University Press.

Clarren, S. K., Alvord, E. C., Sumi, S. M., Streissguth, A. P., & Smith D. W. (1978). Brain malformations related to prenatal exposure to ethanol. *Journal of Pediatrics, 92*, 64-67.

Clarren, S. K., Sampson, P. D., Larsen, J., Donnell, D. J., Barr, H. M., Bookstein, F. L., Martin, D. C., & Streissguth, A. P. (1987). Facial effects of fetal alcohol exposure: Assessment by photographs and morphometric analysis. *American Journal of Medical Genetics, 26*, 651-666.

Clarren, S. K., & Smith, D. W. (1978). The Fetal Alcohol Syndrome. *The New*

England Journal of Medicine, 298(19), 1063-1067.

Clarren, S., & Streissguth, A. (March 1995). Personal Communications.

Coles, C. D., Platzman, K. A., Raskind-Hood, C. L., Brown, R. T., Falek, A., & Smith, I. E. (1997). A comparison of children affected by prenatal alcohol exposure and attention deficit, hyperactivity disorder. *Alcoholism: Clinical and Experimental Research, 21*, 150-161.

Coles, C. D., Smith, I. E., Fernhoff, P. M., & Falek, A. (1985). Neonatal neurobehavioral characteristics as correlates of maternal alcohol use during gestation. *Alcoholism: Clinical and Experimental Research 9*(5), 1-7.

Connors, C. K. (1992) *Manual for the abbreviated symptom questionnnaire*. New York: Multi-health systems.

Conroy, J. W. (1995). *Summary findings: The pennhurst longitudinal study*. Ardmore, PA: The Center For Outcome Analysis.

Conry, J. (1990). Neuropsychological deficits in Fetal Alcohol Syndrome and fetal alcohol effects. *Alcoholism: Clinical and Experimental Research, 14*, 650-655.

Delis, D. C., Kiefner, M., & Fridlund, A. J. (1988). Visuospatial dysfunction following unilateral brain damage: Dissociations in hierarchical and hemispatial analysis. *Journal of Clinical and Experimental Neuropsychology, 10*, 421-431.

Delis, D. C., Kramer, J. H., Kaplan, E., & Ober, B. A. (1994). *Manual for the California verbal learning test-children's version*. San Antonio: Psychological Corporation.

Delis, D. C., Massman, P. J., Butters, N., Salmon, D. P., Shear, P. K., Demadura, T., & Filoteo, J. V. (1992). Spatial cognition in Alzheimer's disease: Subtypes of global-local impairment. *Journal of Clinical and Experimental Neuropsychology, 14*, 463-477.

Diagnostic and statistical manual of mental disorders, 3rd edition (DSM-III). (1987). Washington, D.C.: American Psychiatric Association.

Diagnostic and statistical manual of mental disorders, 4th edition (DSM-IV). (1994). Washington, D.C.: American Psychiatric Association.

Dickerson Mayes, S., Crites, D. L., Bixler, E. O., Humphrey II, F. J., & Mattison, R. E. (1994). Methylphenidate and ADHD: Influence of age, IQ and neurodevelopmental status. *Developmental Medicine and Child Neurology, 36*, 1099-1107.

Douglas, V. I. (1983). Attentional and cognitive problems. In Rutter, M. (Ed.), *Developmental Neuropsychiatry*. (pp. 280-329). New York: Guilford Press.

Driscoll, C. D., Streissguth, A. P., & Riley, E. P. (1990). Prenatal alcohol exposure: Comparability of effects in humans and animal models. *Neurotoxicology and Teratology, 12*, 231-237.

Dunlap, G., Kern-Dunlap, L., Clarke, S., & Robbins, F. R. (1991). Functional assessment, curricular revision, and severe behavior problems. *Journal of Applied Behavior Analysis, 24*, 387-397.

Dunn, L. M., & Dunn, L. M. (1981). *Manual for Peabody Picture Vocabulary Test - Revised*. Circle Pines, MN: American Guidance Service.

Dunst, C. J., Trivette, C. M., & Deal, A. G. (1988). *Enabling and Empowering Families: Principles and Guidelines for Practice*. Cambridge, MA: Brookline Books.

Dyer, K., Alberts, G., & Niemann, G. W. (1995). *Assessment and treatment of an adult with Fetal Alcohol Syndrome: Neuropsychological and behavioral considerations*. Presentation at the Association for Behavior Analysis 22nd Annual Convention, San Francisco, CA.

Ernhart, C. B., Sokol, R. J., Martier, S., Moron, R., Nadler, D., Ager, J. W., & Wolf, A. (1987). Alcohol teratogenicity in the human: A detailed assessment of specificity, critical period, and threshold. *American Journal of Obstetrics and Gynecology, 156*(1), 33-39.

Faustman, E. M., Streissguth, A. P., Stevenson, L. M., Omenn, G. S., & Yoshida, A. (1992). *Role of maternal and fetal alcohol metabolizing genotypes in Fetal Alcohol Syndrome*. Society of Toxicology. 1992 Annual Meeting, Seattle Convention Center, Seattle, Washington.

Finkelstein, N. (1993). Treatment programming for alcohol and drug dependent pregnant women. *International Journal of the Addictions, 28*, 1275–309.

Forrest, F., Florey, C. du V., Taylor, D., McPherson, F., & Young, J. A. (1991). Reported social alcohol consumption during pregnancy and infants' development at 18 months. *British Medical Journal, 303*, 22-26.

Forrest, J. D. (1994). Epidemiology of unintended pregnancy and contraceptive use. *American Journal of Obstetrics and Gynecology, 170*(5), 1485-1489.

Fried, P. A., O'Connell, C. M., & Watkinson, B. (1992). 60- and 72-month follow-up of children prenatally exposed to marijuana, cigarettes, and alcohol: Cognitive and language assessment. *Developmental and Behavioral Pediatrics, 13*, 383-391.

Fried, P. A., & Watkinson, B. (1990). 36- and 48-month neurobehavioral follow-up of children prenatally exposed to marijuana, cigarettes, and alcohol. *Developmental and Behavioral Pediatrics, 11*, 49-58.

Gianoulakis, C. (1990). Rats exposed prenatally to alcohol exhibit impairment in spatial navigation test. *Behavioural Brain Research, 36*, 217-228.

Gillberg, I. C., & Gillberg, C. (1989). Asperger syndrome - some epidemiological considerations: A research note. *Journal of Child Psychology and Psychiatry, 30*, 631-638.

Gold, S., & Sherry, L. (1984). Hyperactivity, learning disabilities and alcohol. *Journal of Learning Disabilities, 17*, 3-6.

Goldstein, G., & Arulanantham, K. (1978). Neural tube defect and renal anomalies in a child with Fetal Alcohol Syndrome. *Journal of Pediatrics, 93*, 636-637.

Goodlett, C. R., Thomas, J. D., & West, J. R. (1991). Long-term deficits in cerebellar growth and rotarod performance of rats following "binge-like" alcohol exposure during the neonatal brain growth spurt. *Neurotoxicology and Teratology, 13,* 69-74.

Graham, J. M., Hanson, J. W., Darby, B. L., Barr, H. M., & Streissguth, A. P. (1988). Independent dsymorphology evaluations a birth and 4 years of age for children exposed to varying amounts of alcohol in utero. *Pediatrics, 81*(6), 722-778.

Grant T. M., Ernst C. C., McAuliff, S., & Streissguth A. P. (1997). The difference game: An assessment tool and intervention strategy for facilitating change in high-risk clients. *Families in Society.*

Grant, T. M., Ernst, C. C., & Streissguth, A. P. (in press) Intervention with high-risk mothers abusing alcohol and drugs: The Seattle Birth to Three advocacy model. *American Journal of Public Health.*

Grant, T. M., Ernst, C. C., Streissguth, A. P., Phipps, P., & Gendler, B. (1996). When case management isn't enough: A model of paraprofessional advocacy for drug- and alcohol-abusing mothers. *Journal of Case Management, 5*(1), 3–11.

Habbick, B. F., Nanson, J. L., Snyder, R. E., Schulman, A., & Casey, R. E. (1996) Fetal alcohol syndrome in Saskatchewan: Unchanged incidence in a 20 year span. *Canadian Journal of Public Health, 87*, 204-208.

Hagerman, R. J. (1996) Bioedical advances in developmental psychology: The case of Fragile-X syndrome. *Developmental Psychology, 32,* 416-424.

Hanson, J. W., Jones, K. L., & Smith, D. W. (1976). Fetal alcohol syndrome: experience with 41 patients. *Journal of the American Medical Association, 235,* 1458-1460.

Hanson, J. W., Streissguth, A. P., & Smith, D. W. (1978). The effects of moderate alcohol consumption during pregnancy on fetal growth and morphogenesis. *Journal of Pediatrics, 92*(3), 457-460

Hartlage, L. C. (1987). Neuropsychology: Definition and history. In L. C. Hartlage, M. J. Asken, & J. L. Hornsby (Eds.), *Essentials of neuropsychological assessment.* New York: Springer Publishing Company.

Hess, J. J., & Niemann, G. W. (1995). *Managing emerging service delivery systems: economic and logistical considerations.* Presentation to Brain Injury Association of America. Annual Meeting: San Diego, CA.

Hynd, G. W., Semrud-Clikeman, M., Lorys, A. R., Novey, E. S., Eliopulos, D., & Lyytinen, H. (1991). Corpus callosum morphology in attention deficit-hyperactivity disorder: Morphometric analysis of MRI. *Journal of Learning Disabilities, 24,* 141-146.

Improving Screening for Fetal Alcohol Syndrome, S. 5688, 54th Legislature, Regular Session, (1995).

Jacobson, S. W., Jacobson, J. L., Sokol, R. J., Martier, S. S., Ager, J. W., & Kaplan-Estrin, M. G. (1993). Teratogenic effects of alcohol on infant development. *Alcoholism: Clinical and Experimental Research, 17*(1), 174-

183.

Janzen, L. A., Nanson, J. L., & Block, G. W. (1994) Neuropsychological Functioning in Preschoolers with FAS. *Neurotoxicology and Teratology, 17*, 3, 273-279.

Janzen, L. A., Nanson, J. L., & Block, G. W. (1995). Neuropsychological evaluation of preschoolers with Fetal Alcohol Syndrome. *Neurotoxicology and Teratology, 17*, 273-379.

Jastak, S., & Wilkinson, G. S. (1984). *Manual for the Wide Range Achievement Test - Revised.* Wilmington, DE: Jastak Associates, Inc.

Jeret, J. S., Serur, D., Wisniewski, K., & Fisch, C. (1986). Frequency of agenesis of the corpus callosum in the developmentally disabled population as determined by computerized tomography. *Pediatric Neuroscience, 12*, 101-103.

Jeret, J. S., Serur, D., Wisniewski, K. E., & Lubin, R. A. (1987). Clinicopathological findings associated with agenesis of the corpus callosum. *Brain Development, 9*, 225-264.

Jones, K. L., & Smith, D. W. (1973). Recognition of the Fetal Alcohol Syndrome in early infancy. *Lancet, 2*, 999-1001.

Jones, K. L., & Smith D. W. (1975). The fetal alcohol syndrome. *Teratology, 12*, 1-10

Jones, K. L., Smith, D. W., Streissguth, A. P., & Myrianthopoulos, N. C. (1974). Outcome in offspring of chronic alcoholic women. *Lancet, 1* (866), 1076-1078.

Jones, K. L., Smith, D. W., Ulleland, C. N., & Streissguth, A. P. (1973). Pattern of malformation in offspring of chronic alcoholic mothers. *Lancet, 1*, 1267-1271.

Kaplan, E., Goodglass, H., & Weintraub, S. (1983). *Boston naming test.* Media, PA: Lea and Febiger.

Kelly, S. J., Goodlett, C. R., Hulsether, S. A., & West, J. R. (1988). Impaired spatial navigation in adult female but not adult male rats exposed to alcohol during the brain growth spurt. *Behavioural Brain Research, 27*, 247-257.

Kleinfeld, J., & Wescott, S. (1993). *Fantastic Antone Succeeds!: Experiences in educating children with fetal alcohol syndrome.* Alaska: University of Alaska Press.

Kodituwakku, P. W., Handmaker, N. S., Cutler, S. K., Weathersby, E. K., & Handmaker, S. D. (1995). Specific impairments in self-regulation in children exposed to alcohol prenatally. *Alcoholism: Clinical and Experimental Research, 19*, 1558-1564.

Koppitz, E. (1971). *The Bender Gestalt Test for Young Children.* New York, NY: Grune and Stratton.

Krogh, C. M. E. (Ed.). (1996). *Compendium of Pharmaceuticals and Specialties (31st ed.).* Ottawa: Canadian Pharmaceutical Association.

Kyllerman, M., Aronson, M., Sabel, K. G., Karlberg, E., Sandin, B., & Olegård, R. (1985). Children of alcoholic mothers: Growth and motor performance compared to matched controls. *Acta Paediatrica Scandinavica, 74*, 20-26.

LaDue, R. A. (1993). *Psychosocial needs associated with Fetal Alcohol Syndrome: practical guidelines for parents and caretakers.* Seattle, WA: University of Washington.

LaDue, R. A., Streissguth, A. P., & Randels, S. P. (1992). Clinical considerations pertaining to adolescents and adults with Fetal Alcohol Syndrome. In T. B. Sonderegger (Ed.), *Perinatal Substance Abuse: Research Findings and Clinical Implications* (pp. 104-131). Baltimore, MD: The Johns Hopkins University Press.

Landesman-Dwyer, S., Keller, L. S., & Streissguth, A. P. (1978). Naturalistic observations of newborns: Effects of maternal alcohol intake. *Alcoholism: Clinical and Experimental Research, 2*, 171-177.

Landesman-Dwyer, S., Ragozin, A. S., & Little, R. E. (1981). Behavioral correlates of prenatal alcohol exposure: A four year follow-up study. *Neurobehavioral Toxicology and Teratology, 3*, 187-193.

Lemoine, P., Harrousseau, H., Borteyru, J. P., & Mennet, J. C. (1968). Les enfants de parents alchooliques. Anomalies observéas. À propos de 127 cas. *Ouest Medical, 21*, 476-482.

Lemoine, P., & Lemoine, P. H. (1992). Avenir des enfants de mères alcooliques (Étude de 105 cas retrouvés à l'âge adulte) et queloques constatations d'intérêt prophylactique [Outcome in the offspring of alcoholic mothers (study of one hundred and five adults) and considerations with a view to prophylaxis]. *Annales de Pediatrie (Paris), 39*, 226-235.

Little, R. E., Streissguth, A. P., & Guzinski, G. M. (1980). Prevention of Fetal Alcohol Syndrome: A model program. *Alcoholism: Clinical and Experimental Research, 4*(2), 185-189.

Majewski, F. (1978). Über schädigende einflüsse des alkohols auf die nachkommen [The damaging effects of alcohol on offspring]. *Der Nervenarzt, 49*, 410-416.

Majewski, F. (1978). Unterzuchungen zur alkohol-embryopathie [Studies on alcohol embryopathy]. *Fortschritte der Medizin, 96*, 2207-2213.

Majewski, F. (1993). Alcohol embryopathy: Experience in 200 patients. *Developmental Brain Dysfunction, 6*, 248-265.

Malbin, D. (1993). *Fetal Alcohol Syndrome and Fetal Alcohol Effects: Strategies for Professionals*. Center City, MN: Hazelden.

Marcus, J. C. (1987). Neurological findings in the Fetal Alcohol Syndrome. *Neuropediatrics, 18*, 158-160.

Mattson, S. N., Gramling, L. S., Delis, D. C., Jones, K. L., & Riley, E. P. (1996) Global - local processing in children prenatally exposed to alcohol. *Child Neuropsychology, 2*, 165-175.

Mattson, S. N., & Riley, E. P. (1996). Brain anomalies in Fetal Alcohol

Syndrome. In: E. L. Abel (Ed.). *Fetal Alcohol Syndrome: From Mechanisms to Prevention*. CRC Press.

Mattson, S. N., & Riley, E. P. (in press). *A review of the neurobehavioral deficits in children with Fetal Alcohol Syndrome or prenatal exposure to alcohol.*

Mattson, S. N., Riley, E. P., Delis, D. C., Stern, C., & Jones, K. L. (1996). Verbal learning and memory in children with Fetal Alcohol Syndrome. *Alcoholism: Clinical and Experimental Research, 20*, 810-816.

Mattson, S. N., Riley, E. P., Gramling, L., Delis, D. C., & Jones, K. L. (in press-a). A neuropsychological comparison of alcohol-exposed children with or without physical features of the Fetal Alcohol Syndrome.

Mattson, S. N., Riley, E. P., Gramling, L., Delis, D. C., & Jones, K. L. (in press-b) Heavy prenatal alcohol exposure leads to IQ deficits with or without physical features of the Fetal Alcohol Syndrome.

Mattson, S. N., Riley, E. P., Jernigan, T. L., Ehlers, C. L., Delis, D. C., Jones, K. L., Stern, C., Johnson, K. A., Hesselink, J. R., & Bellugi, U. (1992). Fetal alcohol syndrome: A case report of neuropsychological, MRI, and EEG assessment of two children. *Alcoholism: Clinical and Experimental Research, 16*, 1001-1003.

Mattson, S. N., Riley, E. P., Jernigan, T. L., Garcia, A., Kaneko, W. M., Ehlers, C. L., & Jones, K. L. (1994). A decrease in the size of the basal ganglia following prenatal alcohol exposure: A preliminary report. *Neurotoxicology and Teratology, 16*, 283-289.

Mattson, S. N., Riley, E. P., Sowell, E. R., Jernigan, T. L., Sobel, D. F., & Jones, K. L. (1996). A decrease in the size of the basal ganglia in children with Fetal Alcohol Syndrome. *Alcoholism: Clinical and Experimental Research, 20*, 1088-1093.

Miller, J. B. (1991). The development of women's sense of self. In: J. D. Jordan, A. G. Kaplan, J. B. Miller, I. P. Stiver, & J. L. Surrey (Eds.). *Women's Growth in Connection* (pp. 11–26). New York, NY: Guilford.

Nanson, J. L. (1990). Behavior in children with Fetal Alcohol Syndrome. In W. I. Fraser (Ed.) *Key Issues in Mental Retardation Research*. London: Blackwell.

Nanson, J. L., & Hiscock, M. (1990). Attention deficits in children exposed to alcohol prenatally. *Alcoholism: Clinical and Experimental Research, 14*, 656-661.

NIAAA. National Institute on Alcohol Abuse and Alcoholism. (1987). *Sixth special report to the U.S. Congress on alcohol and health*. (DHSH Publication No. Adm. 87-1519).

Novick, N. J., & Streissguth, A. P. (1996). Thoughts on treatment of adults and adolescents impaired by Fetal Alcohol Exposure. *Treatment Today, 7*(4), 20-21.

O'Neill, R. E., Horner, R. H., Albin, R. W., Storey, K., & Sprague, J. R. (1990). *Functional Analysis of Problem Behavior: A Practical Assessment Guide.*

Sycamore, IL: Sycamore Press.

Olegård, R., Sabel, K. G., Aronsson, M., Sandin, B., Johansson, P. R., Carlsson, C., Kyllerman, M., Iversen, K., & Hrbek, A. (1979). Effects on the child of alcohol abuse during pregnancy. *Acta Pædiatrica Scandinavica, 275*, 112-121.

Olson, H. C., Feldman, J. J., Streissguth, A. P., & Gonzalez, R. D. (1992). Neuropsychological deficits and life adjustment in adolescents and adults with Fetal Alcohol Syndrome. *Alcoholism: Clinical and Experimental Research, 16*, 380.

Olson, H. C., Sampson, P. D., Barr, H., Streissguth, A. P., & Bookstein, F. L. (1992). Prenatal exposure to alcohol and school problems in late childhood: A longitudinal prospective study. *Development and Psychopathology, 4*, 341-359.

Olson, H. C., Streissguth, A. P, Bookstein, F. L., Barr, H. M., & Sampson, P. D. (1994). Developmental research in behavioral teratology: Effects of prenatal alcohol exposure on child development. In S. L. Friedman & H. C. Haywood (Eds.). *Developmental Follow-Up: Concepts, Domains, and Methods* (pp. 67-112). Orlando, FL: Academic Press.

Parsons, O. A. (1986). Overview of Halstead-Reitan Battery. In T. Incagnoli, G. Goldstein, & C. J. Golden (Eds.). *Clinical Application Of Neuropsychological Test Batteries.* New York: Plenum Press.

Peiffer, J., Majewski, F., Fischbach, H., Bierich, J. R., & Volk, B. (1979). Alcohol embryo- and fetopathy: Neuropathology of 3 children and 3 fetuses. *Journal of the Neurological Sciences, 41*, 125-137.

Pelham, W. E., Harper, G. W., McBurnett, K. Murphy, D. A., Clinton, J., & Thiele, C. (1990). Methylphenidate and baseball playing in ADHD children: Who's on first? *Journal of Consulting and Clinical Psychology, 58*, 130-133.

Pharis, M. E., & Levin, V. S. (1991). "A person to talk to who really cared": High-risk mothers' evaluations of services in an intensive intervention research program. *Child Welfare, LXX* (3), 307-320.

Randall, C.L. (1977). Teratogenic effects of in utero ethanol exposure. In K. Blum, D. Bord, & M. Hamilton (Eds.), *Alcohol and Opiates: Neurochemical and Behavioral Mechanisms* (pp. 91-107). New York: Academic Press.

Raven, J. C., Court, H. L., & Raven, J. (1986). *Manual for the Raven's Progressive Matrices and Vocabulary Scales*. London: Lewis & Co., Ltd.

Raven, J. C., Court, H. L., & Raven, J. (1988). *Manual for the Raven's Progressive Matrices and Vocabulary Scales*. London: Lewis & Co., Ltd.

Reitan, R. M., & Wolfson, D. (1992). *The Halstead-Reitan Neuropsychology Test Battery: Theory and Clinical Interpretation (2nd ed.).* Tucson: Neuropsychology Press.

Reyes, E., Wolfe, J., & Savage, D. D. (1989). The effects of prenatal alcohol exposure on radial arm maze performance in adult rats. *Physiology &*

Behavior, 46, 45-48.

Riley, E. P., Mattson, S. N., Sowell, E. R., Jernigan, T. L., Sobel, D. F., & Jones, K. L. (1995). Abnormalities of the corpus callosum in children prenatally exposed to alcohol. *Alcoholism: Clinical and Experimental Research, 19,* 1198-1202.

Rosett, H. L. (1980). A clinical perspective of the Fetal Alcohol Syndrome. *Alcoholism: Clinical and Experimental Research, 4,* 118.

Rourke, B. P., Bakker, J. L. F., & Strang, J. D. (1983). *Child Neuropsychology: An Introduction to Theory, Research, and Clinical Practice.* New York: Guilford Press.

Russell, M., Czarnecki, D. M., Cowan, R., McPherson, E., & Mudar, P. J. (1991). Measures of maternal alcohol use as predictors of development in early childhood. *Alcoholism: Clinical and Experimental Research, 15,* 991-1000.

Schatzberg, A. F., & Cole, J. O. (1991). *Manual of Clinical Psychopharmacology (2nd ed.).* Washington: American Psychiatric Press.

Shaywitz, S. E., Caparulo, B. K., & Hodgson, E. S. (1981). Developmental language disability as a consequence of prenatal exposure to ethanol. *Pediatrics, 68,* 850-855.

Shaywitz, S. E., Cohen, D. J., & Shaywitz, B. A. (1980). Behavior and learning difficulties in children of normal intelligence born to alcoholic mothers. *The Journal of Pediatrics, 96*(6), 978-982.

Simeon, J.G., & Wiggins, D.M. (1993). Pharmacotherapy of attention-deficit hyperactivity disorder. *Canadian Journal of Psychiatry, 38,* 443-448.

Sokol, R. J., & Clarren, S. K. (1989). Guidelines for use of terminology describing the impact of prenatal alcohol on the offspring. *Alcoholism: Clinical and Experimental Research, 13,* 597-598.

Sowell, E. R., Jernigan, T. L., Mattson, S. N., Riley, E. P., Sobel, D. F., & Jones, K. L. (1996). Abnormal development of the cerebellar vermis in children prenatally exposed to alcohol: Size reduction in lobules I through V. *Alcoholism: Clinical and Experimental Research, 20,* 31-34.

Sparrow, S. S., Bella, D. A., & Cicchetti, D. V. (1984). *Vineland Adaptive Behavior Scales: Interview Edition Survey Form Manual.* Circle Pines, MN: American Guidance Service.

Spohr, H.L., Willms, J., & Steinhausen, H. C. (1993). Prenatal alcohol exposure and long-term developmental consequences. *Lancet, 341*(8850), 907-910.

Spohr, H. L., Willms, J., & Steinhausen, H. C. (1994). The Fetal Alcohol Syndrome in adolescence. *Acta Pediatrica Supplement, 404,* 19-26.

Steinhausen, H. C. (1995). Children of alcoholic mothers: A review. *European Child and Adolescent Psychology, 4*(3). 143-152.

Steinhausen, H. C., Nestler, V., & Spohr, H. L. (1982). Development and psychopathology of children with Fetal Alcohol Syndrome. *Developmental and Behavioral Pediatrics, 3,* 49-54.

Steinhausen, H. C., Willms, J., & Spohr, H. L. (1993). Long-term psychopathological and cognitive outcome of children with Fetal Alcohol Syndrome. *Journal of the American Academy of Child and Adolescent Psychiatry, 32*(5), 990-994.

Steinhausen, H. C., Willms, J., & Spohr, H. L. (1994). Correlates of psychopathology and intelligence in children with Fetal Alcohol Syndrome. *Journal of the American Academy of Child Psychology and Psychiatry, 35,* 323-331.

Stokes, T. F., & Osnes, P. G. (1986). Programming the generalization of children's social behavior. In *Children's Social Behavior, Development, Assessment and Modification.* Orlando, FL: Academic Press.

Stratton, K. R., Howe, C. J., & Battaglia, F. C. (Eds.). (1996). *Fetal Alcohol Syndrome: Diagnosis, epidemiology, prevention, and treatment.* Washington, D.C.: National Academy Press.

Streissguth, A. P. (1992). Fetal alcohol syndrome and fetal alcohol effects: A clinical perspective of later developmental consequences. In I. S. Zagon & T. A. Slotkin (Eds.). *Maternal Substance Abuse and the Developing Nervous System.* San Diego, CA: Academic Press, Inc.

Streissguth, A. P. (1997). *Fetal Alcohol Syndrome: A Guide for Families and Communities.* Baltimore, Maryland: Paul H. Brookes Publishing Co.

Streissguth, A. P., Aase, J. M., Clarren, S. K., Randels, S. P., LaDue, R. A., & Smith, D. F. (1991). Fetal alcohol syndrome in adolescents and adults. *Journal of the American Medical Association, 265*(15), 1961-1967.

Streissguth, A. P., Barr, H. M., Kogan, J., & Bookstein, F. L. (1996). *Understanding the occurrence of secondary disabilities in clients with Fetal Alcohol Syndrome and fetal alcohol effects.* Final Report to the Centers for Disease Control and Prevention (CDC), August, 1996 (Tech. Rep. No. 96-06). Seattle, Washington: University of Washington.

Streissguth, A. P., Barr, H. M., Martin, D. C., & Herman, C. S. (1980). Effects of maternal alcohol, nicotine, and caffeine use during pregnancy on infant mental and motor development at eight months. *Alcoholism: Clinical and Experimental Research, 4*(2), 152-164.

Streissguth, A. P., Barr, H. M., Olson, H. C., Sampson, P. D., Bookstein, F. L., & Burgess, D. M. (1994). Drinking during pregnancy decreases word attack and arithmetic scores on standardized tests: Adolescent data from a population-based prospective study. *Alcoholism: Clinical and Experimental Research, 18,* 248-254.

Streissguth, A. P., Barr, H. M., & Press, S. (1996). A Fetal Alcohol Behavior Scale (FABS) for describing children and adults affected by prenatal alcohol exposure. *Alcoholism: Clinical and Experimental Research, 20*(2), 73a.

Streissguth, A. P., Barr, H. M., & Sampson, P. D. (1990). Moderate prenatal alcohol exposure: Effects on child IQ and learning problems at age 7-1/2 years. *Alcoholism: Clinical and Experimental Research, 14*(5), 662-669.

Streissguth, A. P., Barr, H., Sampson, P. D., & Bookstein, F. L. (1994). Prenatal alcohol and offspring and development: The first fourteen years. *Drug and Alcohol Dependence, 36*, 89-99.

Streissguth, A. P., Barr, H. M., Sampson, P. D., Parrish-Johnson, J. C., Kirchner, G. L., & Martin, D. C. (1986). Attention, distraction and reaction time at age 7 years and prenatal alcohol exposure. *Neurobehavioral Toxicology and Teratology, 8*, 717-725.

Streissguth, A. P., Bookstein, F. L., Sampson, P. D., & Barr, H. M. (1989). Neurobehavioral effects of prenatal alcohol: Part III PLS analyses of neuropsychologic tests. *Neurotoxicology and Teratology, 11*, 493-507.

Streissguth, A. P., Bookstein, F. L., Sampson, P. C., & Barr, H. M. (1993). *The Enduring Effects of Prenatal Alcohol Exposure on Child Development: Birth through Seven Years, a Partial Least Squares Solution.* Ann Arbor, MI: University of Michigan Press.

Streissguth, A. P., Clarren, S. K., & Jones, K. L. (1985). Natural history of the fetal alcohol syndrome: A 10-year follow-up of eleven patients. *Lancet, 13*. 85-91.

Streissguth, A. P., Grant, T. M., Barr, H. M., Brown, Z. A., Martin, J. C., Mayock, D. E., Ramey, S. L., & Moore, L. (1991). Cocaine and the use of alcohol and other drugs during pregnancy. *American Journal of Obstetrics & Gynecology, 164*(5), 1239-1243.

Streissguth, A. P., Herman, C. S., & Smith, D. W. (1978). Intelligence, behavior, and dysmorphogenesis in the Fetal Alcohol Syndrome: A report on 20 patients. *Journal of Pediatrics, 92*(3), 363-367.

Streissguth, A. P., Herman, C. S., & Smith, D. W. (1978). Stability of intelligence in the Fetal Alcohol Syndrome: A preliminary report. *Alcoholism: Clinical and Experimental Research, 2*(2), 165-170.

Streissguth, A. P., LaDue, R. A., & Randels, S. P. (1986). *A Manual on Adolescents and Adults with Fetal Alcohol Syndrome with Special Reference to American Indians.* Seattle, WA: University of Washington.

Streissguth A. P., LaDue R. A., & Randels S. P. (1988). *A Manual on Adolescents and Adults with Fetal Alcohol Syndrome with Special Reference to American Indians (2nd ed).* Albuquerque, NM: Indian Health Service.

Streissguth, A. P., Martin, D. C. Barr, H. M., Sandman, B. M., Kirschner, G. L., & Darby, B. L. (1984). Intrauterine alcohol and nicotine exposure: Attention and reaction time in 4 year old children. *Developmental Psychology, 20*, 553-541.

Streissguth, A. P., & Randels, S. (1988). Long term effects of Fetal Alcohol Syndrome. In Robinson, G. C., & Armstrong, R. W. (Eds.) *Alcohol and Child/Family Health.* (pp. 135- 147). Vancouver, B. C., Canada: University of British Columbia.

Streissguth, A. P., Randels, S. P., & Smith, D. F. (1991). A test-retest study of intelligence in patients with the Fetal Alcohol Syndrome: Implications for care. *Journal of the American Academy of Child and Adolescent Psychiatry*, *30*(4), 584-587.

Streissguth, A. P., & Rohsenow, D. J. (1974). *Intellectual Development in Offspring of Chronic Alcoholic Mothers and Matched Controls*. Paper presented at Western Psychological Association Meeting, San Francisco.

Streissguth A. P., Sampson P. D., & Barr H. M. (1989). Neurobehavioral dose-response effects of prenatal alcohol exposure in humans from infancy to adulthood. *Annals of the New York Academy of Sciences*, (562). 145-158.

Streissguth, A. P., Sampson, P. D., Olson, H. C., Bookstein, F. L., Barr, H. M., Scott, M., Feldman, J., & Mirsky, A. F. (1994). Maternal drinking during pregnancy: Attention and short-term memory in 14 year old offspring — a longitudinal prospective study. *Alcoholism: Clinical and Experimental Research, 18*, 202-218.

Surgeon General's advisory on alcohol and pregnancy. (1981). *FDA Drug Bulletin, 11*(2). Rockville, Maryland: Department of Health and Human Services.

Surrey, J. L. (1991). The "self-in-relation": A theory of women's development (pp. 51-66). In: J. D. Jordan, A. G. Kaplan, J. B. Miller, I. P. Stiver, & J. L. Surrey (Eds.). *Women's Growth in Connection*. New York, NY: Guilford.

Swanson, J. M., Barlow, A., & Kinsboutne, M. (1981). Task specificity of responses to stimulant drugs in laboratory tests. In M. Gittmen (Ed.). *Strategic Interventions for Hyperactive Children*. Armonk, N. Y.: M. E. Sharpe.

Tenbrinck, M. S. & Buchin, S. Y. (1975). Fetal alcohol syndrome: Report of a case. *Journal of the American Medical Association, 232*, 1144-1147.

Tirosh, E., Sadeh, A., Munvez, R., & Lavie, P. (1993). Effects of methylphenidate on sleep in children with attention-deficit hyperactivity disorder. *American Journal of Diseases of Children, 147*, 1313-1315.

Uecker, A., & Nadel, L. (1996). Spatial locations gone awry: Object and spatial memory deficits in children with Fetal Alcohol Syndrome. *Neuropsychologia, 34*, 209-233.

Wechsler, D. (1967). *WPPSI Manual: Wechsler Preschool and Primary Scale of Intelligence*. New York: The Psychological Corporation.

Wechsler, D. (1974). *Manual for the Wechsler Intelligence Scale for Children, Revised*. San Antonio: Psychological Corporation.

Wechsler, D. (1974). *WISC-R Wechsler Intelligence Scale for Children, Revised*. New York: The Psychological Corporation.

Wechsler, D. (1981). *WAIS-R Manual: Wechsler Adult Intelligence Scale – Revised*. New York: The Psychological Corporation.

Wechsler, D. (1989). *Manual for the Wechsler Preschool and Primary Scale of Intelligence - Revised*. San Antonio: Psychological Corporation.

Wilsnack, S. C., Wilsnack, R. W., & Hiller-Sturnhofel S. (1994). How women drink: Epidemiology of women's drinking and problem drinking. *Alcohol Health and Research World, 18*(3), 173-81.

Wisniewski, K., Dambska, M., Sher, J. H., & Qazi, Q. (1983). A clinical neuropathological study of the Fetal Alcohol Syndrome. *Neuropediatrics, 14,* 197-201.

Authors' Affiliations

Gregory Alberts, Ph.D. • Chief Neuropsychologist, Bancroft, Inc., Haddonfield, New Jersey

Marita Aronson, Ph.D. • Psychologist, Department of Pediatrics, East Hospital, University of Göteborg, Göteborg, Sweden

Susan Astley, Ph.D. • Assistant Professor of Epidemiology and Pediatrics, Children's Hospital and Medical Center, University of Washington School of Medicine, Seattle, Washington

The Honorable Judge C. C. Barnett • Provincial Court of British Columbia, Williams Lake, British Columbia

Helen Barr, M.S., M.A. • Database Manager and Biostatistician, Fetal Alcohol & Drug Unit, Department of Psychiatry and Behavioral Sciences, University of Washington School of Medicine, Seattle, Washington

Gerald Block, M.S. • Research Assistant, Alvin Buckwold Child Development Program, Royal University Hospital, Saskatoon, Saskatchewan

Fred Bookstein, Ph.D. • Distinguished Research Scientist, Institute of Gerontology, University of Michigan, Ann Arbor, Michigan

Sterling Clarren, M.D. • Professor of Pediatrics and Director, FAS Diagnostic Clinic, University of Washington School of Medicine, Seattle, Washington

Jeanice Dagher-Margosian, J.D. • Criminal Defense Attorney, Ann Arbor, Michigan

Jocie DeVries • Executive Director and Parent Advocate, FAS Family Resource Institute, Lynnwood, Washington

Michael Dorris • Author, *The Broken Cord*

235

Thomas Dunne, M.S.W. • Social Worker, Society of Counsel Representing Accused Persons, Seattle, Washington

Kathleen Dyer, Ph.D. • Director, Evaluation, Research and Staff Development, Bancroft, Inc., Haddonfield, New Jersey

Cara Ernst, M.A. • Program Evaluator, Birth to 3 Program, Fetal Alcohol & Drug Unit, Department of Psychiatry and Behavioral Sciences, University of Washington School of Medicine, Seattle, Washington

Therese Grant, Ph.C. • Director, Birth to 3 Project, Fetal Alcohol & Drug Unit, Department of Psychiatry and Behavioral Sciences, University of Washington School of Medicine, Seattle, Washington

Joseph J. Hess, Jr., M.S.W., M.B.A. • Executive Vice President, Bancroft, Inc., Haddonfield, New Jersey

Richard Jackson, M.D., M.P.H. • Director, National Center for Environmental Health, Centers for Disease Control and Prevention, Atlanta, Georgia

Jonathan Kanter, M.A. • Research Assistant, Behavioral Research & Therapy Clinics, Psychology Department, University of Washington, Seattle, Washington

Julia Kogan, Ed.M. • Project Director, CDC Project, Fetal Alcohol & Drug Unit, Department of Psychiatry and Behavioral Sciences, University of Washington School of Medicine, Seattle, Washington

Robin LaDue, Ph.D. • Clinical Assistant Professor, Department of Psychiatry and Behavioral Sciences, University of Washington, Seattle, Washington

Mike Lowry • Governor, Washington State, 1992-1996

Jan Lutke • Executive Director, FAS/E Support Network of British Columbia, Surrey, British Columbia

Sarah N. Mattson, Ph.D. • Psychologist, Center for Behavioral Teratology, San Diego State University, San Diego, California

Peter H. D. McKee, J.D. • Attorney, Theiler, Douglas, Drachler, & McKee, Seattle, Washington

Jo Nanson, Ph.D. • Psychologist, Alvin Buckwold Child Development Program, Royal University Hospital, Saskatoon, Saskatchewan

George W. Niemann, Ph.D. • President and Chief Executive Officer, Bancroft, Inc., Haddonfield, New Jersey

Natalie Novick, Ph.D. • Clinical Psychologist, Mountlake Terrace, Washington

Jennifer K. Porter, B.A. • Medical Student, Fetal Alcohol & Drug Unit, Department of Psychiatry and Behavioral Sciences, University of Washington School of Medicine, Seattle, Washington

Edward P. Riley, Ph.D. • Director, Center for Behavioral Teratology, San Diego State University, San Diego, California

Claire Anita Schmucker • Private Case Manager, Seattle, Washington

Jill Snyder • Honors Student, Psychology, University of Saskatchewan, Saskatoon, Saskatchewan

Richard Snyder, M.D. • Alvin Buckwold Child Development Program, Department of Pediatrics, Royal University Hospital, Saskatoon, Saskatchewan

Ann Streissguth, Ph.D. • Director, Fetal Alcohol & Drug Unit, Department of Psychiatry and Behavioral Sciences, University of Washington School of Medicine, Seattle, Washington

Patricia Tanner-Halverson, Ph.D. • FAS/FAE Project Director, Tohono O'Odham Reservation, Sells, Arizona

Ann Waller, M.Ed. • Executive Assistant, FAS Family Resource Institute, Lynnwood, Washington

Thomas Wentz, Ph.D. • Assistant Professor, Special Education, Loras College, Dubuque, Iowa

Author Index

Subject Index

Italic *t* refers to tables; *f* refers to figures.